The ADD Nutrition Solution

The ADD Nutrition Solution

A Drug-Free Thirty-Day Plan

MARCIA ZIMMERMAN, C.N.

AN OWL BOOK
Henry Holt and Company | New York

Henry Holt and Company, LLC
Publishers since 1866
115 West 18th Street
New York, New York 10011

Henry Holt® is a registered trademark of
Henry Holt and Company, LLC.

Library of Congress Cataloging-in-Publication Data
Zimmerman, Marcia.
    The ADD nutrition solution: a drug-free thirty-day plan /
Marcia Zimmerman.—1st ed.
        p.   cm.
    Includes index.
    ISBN 0-8050-6128-2
    1. Attention-deficit hyperactivity disorder—Popular works.
    2. Attention-deficit hyperactivity disorder—Nutritional aspects.
    3. Attention-deficit-disordered children.   I. Title.
    RJ506.H9Z   1999   98-45420
    616.85'890654—dc21   CIP

Henry Holt books are available for special promotions and
premiums. For details contact: Director, Special Markets.

First Edition 1999

Designed by Kelly Soong Too

Printed in the United States of America

10   9   8   7

The information contained in this book is intended to inform and educate. There is no claim
being made for the diagnosis, cure, treatment, or prevention of disease, nor should these recommendations take the place of medical advice. The nutritional therapies recommended in this
book should be guided by your physician.

To Sean Michael with my love.
Love brings hope, trust, and understanding
You are a beautiful and talented person.

CONTENTS

ACKNOWLEDGMENTS

The ADD Nutrition Solution has been a collective effort. My husband, Jon Zimmerman, has spent hours editing and formatting the book. My nutritionist colleague Carolyn Martinez has been tireless in her pursuit of products for your shopping cart, and she scrutinized hundreds of labels for offending ingredients. My nutrition associate Karla Schmidt "kid tested" dozens of recipes and analyzed them for nutritional content. Terry Zeyen from the UCLA Bio-Med Library scoured hundreds of papers, medical journals, and medical books, doing the scientific discovery for this book.

Special thanks go as well to my friend Jean Carper, my agent Jenny Bent, and my editor Amelia Sheldon, who have tirelessly helped me navigate the journey to publishing my first book; and to Nature's Way of Springville, Utah, without whose help and encouragement this book could not have been written.

When Marcia Zimmerman told me she was writing a book on attention deficit disorder and how to handle it through nutrition, I knew her book would be unique, for she brings to the subject years of lecturing, studying, and recommending diets that have helped countless children and adults overcome this misunderstood phenomenon.

I first met Marcia several years ago after one of her lectures in Baltimore and recognized that she was a first-rate educator as well as an expert in nutrition and the formulation of nutritional supplements. She is well versed in the chemistry of the body, which makes her extremely well qualified to speak out and give sober, nonhysterical advice on this troublesome disorder and, most important, a well-thought-out day-to-day practical plan, which at long last may help erase the *underlying causes* of ADD, not just its symptoms.

New scientific findings endorse this approach. Scientists now increasingly recognize that the brain is mightily influenced by nutritional factors. At a September 1998 conference at the National Institutes of Health in Bethesda, Maryland, on omega-3 fatty acids and the brain, researchers from all over the world reported the latest findings on how eating particular types of fat affected the neurological system. Both Marcia and I attended. Speaker after speaker tied a lack of essential fatty acids, including omega-3 fish-oil type oils, to errors in brain metabolism and information processing. The result: increased vulnerability to depression, schizophrenia, learning disabilities, dyslexia, and ADD. There was evidence that replenishing the fatty acids could correct certain deficiencies within brain cells, leading to improvement in symptoms and, in some cases, changes in the brain itself as verified by sophisticated brain imaging.

It is sobering to realize how dependent the brain is on the "right foods" at all stages of life and how critical nutrition is in shaping the structure and workings of the brain of a fetus as well as of a young child. Such sustenance, research shows, helps determine mental functioning, including intelligence, attention, concentration, problem-solving, and memory.

At the same time, one senses a new growing dissatisfaction with the way ADD is medically treated in this country, mainly with Ritalin. At a November 1998 NIH "consensus" conference on treating ADD, some psychiatrists raised their voices against the wholesale and perhaps lifelong use of strong stimulants, such as Ritalin, by children and adults. They argue, as does Marcia Zimmerman, that this drug does not address the real cause of ADD and may, in fact, cause irreparable harm.

In any event, Marcia Zimmerman's *ADD Nutrition Solution* is a much needed and sensible answer to one of the nation's most alarming and fast-growing problems. Anyone who needs help with this disorder should give her advice a try. The one-month trial it takes to find out if it works could make a monumental difference in the life of a child or an adult.

JEAN CARPER

Attention Deficit/Hyperactivity Disorder (AD/HD) is the fastest growing childhood disorder in the United States. According to information
published in the *Journal of the American Academy of Child and Adolescent
Psychiatry* in November 1996, an astounding 5 to 7 percent of American
children and teens, approximately four million by 1999, are believed to
suffer from attention deficits. In some areas of the country, about half of
all students are labeled as victims of this mentally disabling disorder. In
addition, another thirteen million adults are believed to suffer from
AD/HD, bringing the total to a staggering seventeen million Americans
who battle this condition daily. The rapid spread of AD/HD has been
called an "epidemic."

"With the exception of AIDS, there are few examples of such a rapid
epidemic spread of a serious condition in recent years," Gene Haislip,
former administrator of the U.S. Drug Enforcement Agency, said in a
DEA address in December 1996.

Many parents I've talked to find these facts confusing and troubling.
Are we labeling our children AD/HD simply because it is a convenient
way to put down natural creativity and exuberance, or is there a real

medical condition that we can prevent or address? As you may imagine, the answer is not a simple one.

AD/HD is a valid disorder; ask parents who have a child with the properly diagnosed condition and they will immediately agree. Adults who have been diagnosed with AD/HD, based largely upon symptoms dating from childhood, find comfort in knowing there really is a medical reason why they have had such a difficult time managing their lives. However, we have adopted a somewhat cavalier attitude toward this disorder in the 1990s, regarding it as a natural by-product of the social and environmental climate today. We almost make a joke of it, using it as a handy label for behavior that is unusual or even bizarre. Most of us have times when we think we have attention deficits, as if the condition exists within each of us, but we learn to overcome it. However, this is not so.

Attention deficit disorders are serious neurological conditions that can result in severe behavioral dysfunction. The American Psychiatric Association (APA) has compiled a list of symptoms most commonly associated with different types of AD/HD. Two sets of criteria, one for the AD/HD-inattentive type formerly called ADD, and the other for the AD/HD-hyperactive/impulsive type, have been published by APA in the fourth edition of the *Diagnostic and Statistical Manual of Mental Disorders (DSM IV)*. These criteria are used by doctors to help identify those suspected of having the problem, and because they are listed in an official publication of psychiatric disorders, represent a serious diagnosis with potentially grave consequences.

Important Facts About AD/HD:

- AD/HD is the most commonly diagnosed psychiatric condition found among young people
- AD/HD affects 5 to 10 percent of school-age children according to top scientists. As much as 7 percent of the earth's population may have AD/HD—a total of 399 million, more than the combined populations of the United States, Mexico, and Canada
- In some areas of the country, about half of all children in schools have been diagnosed with AD/HD

Considerable confusion exists over what to call attention deficits. The American Psychiatric Association in 1994 re-classified the several forms of attention deficits as *Attention Deficit Hyperactive Disorders*. Subtypes that are recognized include *inattentive*, *hyperactive*, and *impulsive*. An individual can have any one of the subtypes or a *combined* type.

However, the most recognizable term is still ADD, which identifies all of the syndromes, and that is what I have chosen to use in this book's title. While most professionals refer to ADD or ADHD when distinguishing inattentive and hyperactive elements, they generally use a generic ADD/HD, ADD/H or AD/HD when writing about the disorders. I have chosen to go this route (AD/HD) in discussing the disorders within the text of this book.

The treatment most often recommended for alleviating AD/HD symptoms is stimulant medication, and the most commonly prescribed drug for the condition is methylphenidate (Ritalin). Very young children are often put on this medication and continue to use it for years. According to the National Institutes of Health, the National Institutes of Mental Health, the Public Health Service, and the U.S. Department of Health and Human Services, 80 percent of the children prescribed it at a young age will continue to need this medication as adolescents and 50 percent will need to continue its use into adulthood. Moreover, the United States consumes five times more Ritalin than the rest of the planet, according to U.S. Drug Enforcement Agency sources. Consumption of Ritalin has grown over 600 percent since the early 1990s and continues to grow despite rigid DEA controls over the annual amount that can be produced, aimed at curbing potential abuse.

It seems odd that a stimulant can calm down a hyperactive person. But it makes sense if you consider that faulty wiring in the brain is thought to be a major cause of AD/HD symptoms and that Ritalin and other stimulants can effectively "jump start" the brain, bypassing short circuits and clarifying messages sent between brain cells. However, the effects of such prescriptions tend to be very short-term, leading to the need for medication every three or four hours. This explains why long lines of children waiting outside school nurses' offices are a common sight in many parts of the country. By lunchtime, the child's morning dose of Ritalin has worn off, and he or she needs a refresher dose in order to make it through the afternoon. Not only are the effects of stimulant medications short-term, they provide no long-term relief because they do not repair the underlying chemical problem, but merely alleviate its symptoms.

What if there was a way to not suppress, but actually overcome attention deficits without the use of drugs? *The ADD Nutrition Solution* does just that. In this book I examine the history of research on AD/HD and the effects of diet on brain and nervous function. I will also present the latest findings of sophisticated neuro-imaging techniques that reveal how dietary change and use of select nutritional supplements can repair faulty brain circuitry to help AD/HD sufferers of any age sharpen their ability to learn and to increase concentration, focus, and memory. I will show you how to identify the foods that are contributing to your own or your child's problem, how to substitute better choices, and how to balance brain function by choosing when to eat specific groups of foods depending on whether you wish to optimize alertness or promote sleepiness. I have designed a simple systematic approach to diet modification by showing you what you should and shouldn't stock in your cupboard, what foods are most commonly associated with behavioral problems, and how to fix exciting meals that will alleviate AD/HD symptoms. Finally, I will tell you how supplementing your diet before and during pregnancy can optimize the mental health of your child.

NUTRITION IS THE ANSWER

If you make a point of educating your child on the importance of nutrition in addressing AD/HD, you will most likely find that he or she learns easily and, with encouragement, will use this information to take responsibility for a lifetime of his or her own health and well-being. Whether you as an adult use this plan alone or combine it with medication, you will be improving brain function and increasing your ability to focus and process information.

As I share the long-term, drug-free approach to AD/HD, I will introduce you to some people who feel they have greatly benefited from the thirty-day nutrition and supplement plan. I hope that this program and its explanation will be as helpful to you and your family as it has been for them.

The ADD Nutrition Solution

PART I

Are Attention Deficit Disorders the Plague of the Nineties?

When he was expected to use his mind,
he felt like a right-handed person
who has to do something with his left.

—Georg Christoph Lichtenberg

Do I or My Child Have an Attention Deficit Disorder?

What are attention deficits exactly and how do you know if you are suffering from them? These are the first questions we must address before discussing treatment of ADD. To do so, let's take a quick look at the history of this condition and the evolution of its definition and diagnosis.

Attention deficits have evolved over the years in the terminology used and the classification of the symptoms. The latest revisions to the disorders are defined in the *Diagnostic and Statistical Manual of Mental Disorders*, fourth edition, or *DSM IV*. Currently all attention deficits are grouped under the designation AD/HD or attention deficit/hyperactive disorder. Two main categories of AD/HD are defined, AD/HD predominantly *inattentive* and AD/HD predominantly *hyperactive-impulsive*. A third category is considered, AD/HD-*combined*, that is, a combination of inattentive and hyperactive or impulsive types. For all three types, the condition must have persisted for at least six months, and have occurred before the age of seven, in order to be identified as a true attention deficit disorder. The adult condition is diagnosed by examining childhood history, interviewing parents and others who knew the individual as a child, plus evaluating the adult symptoms.

THE AD/HD-INATTENTIVE TYPE

AD/HD-*inattentive* describes the child or adult who has trouble paying attention, completing assignments, frequently daydreams, and is easily distracted. This classification has replaced the older term "ADD," although most professionals still call the condition ADD.

Many AD/HD-inattentive children are quick learners and are easily bored. They need fast-paced activities to keep them engaged. Others with attention problems respond well to a structured environment both at home and at school. We can assist these children with learning by providing more structure so they are comfortable and know what to expect.

AD/HD Behaviors

INATTENTIVE	HYPERACTIVE/IMPULSIVE
Difficulty Organizing Tasks—Can't Get Started	Talks Too Much
Mental Restlessness—Constant Brain Chatter	Difficulty Doing Tasks Alone
Easily Distracted—Attention Easily Diverted	Physical Restlessness—Finger Tapping, Leg Restlessness
Difficulty Completing Tasks	Engages in Physically Daring Activities
Shifts from One Task to Another	Always on the Go, As If Driven by a Motor
Difficulty Sustaining Attention—Can't Focus	Impulsive
Doesn't Appear to Listen to Others	Often Interrupts Others
Constantly Loses Possessions	Impatient
Forgets Easily—Can't Remember "To Do's"	Unpredictable Behavior
Trouble Keeping Track of Events—Sequence	Hot and Explosive Temper

(adapted from *DSM IV* criteria)

Adults with the inattentive type of AD/HD function best when they resist the tendency to procrastinate, which is one of their worst problems. Being extremely forgetful, absentminded, and unorganized are other characteristics of the adult disorder. Many adults have learned to overcome these problems by instituting structured procedures into everything they do. They often find they accomplish most when they work from detailed to-do lists, and counteract forgetfulness with procedures such as designating a specific place to store keys when not in use. They often choose professions that require quick decision making and physical activity over those that require intense concentration for long periods of time. Others develop a technique known as "hyperfocus" that allows them to shut out all distractions around them in order to accomplish tasks.

THE AD/HD-HYPERACTIVE/IMPULSIVE TYPE

AD/HD-*hyperactive/impulsive* individuals are always on the go and tend to be unpredictable, impatient, hot tempered, and impulsive. They can, however, maintain attention for long periods of times, especially if engaged in something that interests them. Children with this type of attention deficit often find computer-based activities engaging, interesting, and self-instructing; others do well in sports, dance, gymnastics, or music. Giving them opportunities to explore these kinds of activities can be quite helpful.

Adults with this kind of AD/HD can have trouble with relationships, both in their personal lives and in careers. This is because they often resent authority of any kind. They often choose business entrepreneurship, which allows them more flexibility and use of their talents than other work models. Change for this group of individuals is often welcomed, although they can also be fanatics about order.

THE AD/HD-COMBINED TYPE

AD/HD-*combined* refers to the children, or occasionally the adults, who are inattentive, impulsive, and hyperactive. They can have any of the symptoms included in the other two groups. They are often described as those who talk too much, constantly distract others, butt into conversations, do not wait their turn, are forgetful, lack responsibility, and are unable to follow instructions or get along with peers. They have the greatest difficulty fitting into the mainstream of life and are extremely resistant to change. As a result, these individuals are most likely to have learning difficulties, defiant behavior, and developmental disorders along with AD/HD.

DSM IV categorization of the disorders may seem quite clear, and you may have already been trying to decide whether any of these descriptions fit you or your child. However, getting AD/HD diagnosed can be confusing and frustrating, especially for parents. Not only is it devastating to discover your child has a disability, but finding out the exact nature of the child's condition can be elusive.

DIAGNOSING AD/HD

Amazingly, a variety of doctors applying *DSM IV* criteria to evaluate the same child will often arrive at different conclusions. Each observer brings his or her own judgment to the diagnosis and there are no standard or "normal" levels of activity upon which to base comparisons. A physician must determine whether your child's behavior is extreme or inappropriate for his age, and professional opinions can vary for many reasons, including which area of the country the child comes from! Areas of the United States with the greatest incidence of AD/HD are the Great Lakes region, the upper East Coast, and the southeast and southern regions. Regional influences do seem to affect the diagnosis, for reasons that are as yet unclear. Interestingly enough, however, we find the areas of greatest incidence of AD/HD overlap those of highest concentration of nitrates and phosphates from long-term agricultural and industrial applications. Add to this the fact that attention deficits are actually a cluster of symptoms, and every diagnosis will differ in at least one aspect. In the end, many parents are frustrated and angry because they cannot get a simple answer: Does my child have an attention deficit disorder . . . and if so, what kind? What, then, should you look for in an accurate diagnosis of AD/HD?

MEDICAL REVIEW

A diagnosis for this disorder should be given only after a thorough evaluation by a team of professionals who specialize in AD/HD. First, you should see a pediatrician to rule out possible medical reasons for the disorder. AD/HD will not reveal itself through the usual battery of laboratory tests, although some abnormalities in brain function have been observed with the use of brain-imaging techniques such as magnetic resonance imaging (MRI) and positron emission tomography (PET) scans. "There is no laboratory test or set of tests that currently can be used to make a definitive diagnosis," according to Dennis Cantwell, M.D., *Journal of the American Academy of Child and Adolescent Psychiatry*, August 1996. These techniques to determine faulty brain function are rarely used with children, however, because little is known about the relationship between observed abnormalities and symptoms.

HISTORY AND OBSERVATION

Parents or care-givers are really the only ones who can provide specific evidence that a child had AD/HD tendencies before he or she entered school. Parents often notice different behavior patterns in their child from birth. However, AD/HD behavior usually becomes most noticeable to parents and teachers in children between the ages of three and four, and is often seen when a child is placed in preschool.

Teacher observations are important in helping to define the specific kind of AD/HD a child has because of his or her ability to make comparisons with a child's peers to determine age-appropriate behavior. The teacher also has evidence of the child's performance or lack of it, through handwriting samples and workbooks. Teachers are constantly evaluating a child's work habits, off-task behaviors, responsibility, and social skills. Oftentimes a teacher is the first to suspect a child has AD/HD and may seek assistance from the school psychologist to help evaluate the child.

Next, a professional team that usually includes a psychiatrist or psychologist and a therapist performs a battery of tests. They obtain information from standard questionnaires about the child's behavior that are filled out by the child's parents and teacher. The psychiatric team also observes the child either in the classroom or in an observation area at a medical center.

Following observation, they test the child to measure his ability to sustain attention, his I.Q., and his learning rate. The tests and parental observations are then evaluated by the team of professionals who collectively agree on a definitive diagnosis. Currently there are no standard tests for the adult disorder, which is diagnosed by current symptoms, interviews, and childhood history.

DIAGNOSTIC TESTS

Diagnostic tests for children typically include Connor's parent and teacher rating scales, which rank a child's behavior based on *DSM IV* criteria. Parents should be aware that behaviors of an ADD child mentioned in Connor's include: doesn't appear to listen, loses things a lot, fails to do things, throws temper tantrums, and instigates physical abuse toward siblings or parents. For teachers, the behaviors an ADD child might show in school include off-task behavior, leaving his/her seat, interrupting others, and shifting from one task to another. The more infractions a child commits, the higher the score, with a score of 48 the highest possible. Fifteen is considered the point at which AD/HD is suggested.

The Test of Variables of Attention or TOVA measures learning aptitude in children and adults. This non-language-based test measures a person's ability to complete tasks, concentrate for periods of time, and make connections between concepts. It is often used to determine if learning disabilities exist. Both the Connor and TOVA tests are easy to administer and are often used to assess results in clinical trials.

Additional tests include the Child Behavior Checklist for parents and teachers, and the newest test based on *DSM IV* criteria, the Attention-Deficit/Hyperactivity Disorder Test, or AD/HDT. This test helps categorize AD/HD individuals aged three to twenty-three years and can be completed by parents, teachers, and other professionals. There are separate tests for males and females, since the behaviors between the sexes are quite different.

Dr. Paul Wender, from the University of Utah, has developed a test that is used to identify adults who have lingering symptoms from an AD/HD condition in childhood. This test is called the Utah Criteria for the Diagnosis of AD/HD–Residual Type. Dr. Russell Barkley, an expert in adult AD/HD, has also developed a detailed, structured interview that is often used to identify the adult disorder. Both tests are important in identifying AD/HD in adults, since no standardized tests are available.

If your child has been through an ADD testing process more than once, you may have been given different versions of the AD/HD diagnosis. This is common. Don't be discouraged if this has been your experience. For our purposes it doesn't matter which form of AD/HD your child has or even if he has a *mild undiagnosed* case of the disorder; whatever situation you face, my *30-Day Plan* will help curtail AD/HD symptoms because with it we are addressing the underlying nutritional needs of the brain. If you are a parent just trying to improve your child's behavior or quiet it a bit, the suggestions here will be equally effective.

WHAT SHOULD YOU LOOK FOR?

One of the more common tip-offs to parents that their child might be AD/HD is that they've always noticed that their child behaves differently from others his/her age. Edward Hallowell, M.D., and John Ratey, M.D., Boston psychiatrists and authors of *Driven to Distraction*, emphasize that AD/HD behavior is characterized by comparison with a group of peers. Among others his own age the AD/HD child is *markedly more impulsive, restless, and inattentive*. AD/HD is different from "high energy." It is a more intense pattern of behavior that must have *persisted for at least six months, occurred before the age of seven, and set the child's actions apart from others' his age*. When I discussed the diagnosis with Dr. Ratey in June 1998, he emphasized that to be truly characterized as AD/HD, *the behaviors must be severe enough to be disabling*.

Observation of these behaviors is often what compels parents to check out AD/HD as a possible cause. They first suspect AD/HD when it is evident that their three-year-old's behavior is unlike that of other children his or her age. Often, they note that the child was "different" from birth. The family case study I will present in chapter 2 clearly illustrates this point. Observations such as these are extremely valuable in arriving at a diagnosis of AD/HD, because they involve behaviors only the parents may have observed. Most experts agree that the earlier a child is identified as AD/HD, the better. However, they caution that use of medication in response to such a diagnosis in a child under age six is unwarranted and not proven to be beneficial.

A child's first three years are the most critical in his or her development of healthy self-esteem. Early detection of problem behaviors gives parents the chance to work on any emotional and learning issues effectively that arise along with ADD in their child. Therapies, such as nutrition and behavior modification, are better utilized at this early age as well. Nutrition is the best therapy you can use for your preschool child, whether he or she is AD/HD or not. Healthy eating habits can easily be taught to young children. Their young brains are easily molded by good nutrients, but they can just as easily be disrupted by harmful ones like hydrogenated fats and additives. I will show you why this is the case and guide you through the process of dietary change.

AD/HD does occur in very small children, and they are often our brightest and most promising youth. Many AD/HD-diagnosed children have been considered below average in intelligence, and we have to be extremely careful that AD/HD children do not get the idea that they are stupid or slow. Parents, seeking to avoid this stigma, come to their AD/HD child's defense by describing him or her as having a "different learning style." This approach is fine, but if we truly believe it, we must provide some accommodation for these differences. Parents often find themselves battling for their child's right to an educational style that fits his or her needs. If the public education system cannot meet these special needs, parents may need to consider private, charter, or home schooling.

"PURE" AD/HD RARELY EXISTS!

Diagnosis of AD/HD is often complicated by the presence of other conditions that coexist or are *comorbid* with AD/HD. The most common are learning disabilities, including poor visual perception, auditory-language dysfunction, and poor memory and/or communication skills. As a result, the AD/HD child with learning disabilities may be assigned to special education classes.

Neuropathological disorders that typically coexist with AD/HD are autism, oppositional defiant disorder, and pervasive developmental disorder. These conditions dramatically affect the outcome and treatment of the AD/HD individual. We are just beginning to link these coexisting conditions with dysfunctions in specific areas of the brain. As more is learned about coexisting conditions, better treatment strategies can be planned. Nutrition is the common thread that runs through all of them, however, and a specific dietary plan should be part of any treatment.

Allergies are extremely common in AD/HD individuals, both children and adults. Allergies cause disruption in brain function, and minimizing their effects is so important in overcoming AD/HD that I have devoted a detailed explanation on how they affect the condition in chapter 8. Although allergies are a common problem in those with AD/HD, each victim of this mysterious disabling condition will have his or her own set of symptoms. That's why parents will say "my child has *an* attention deficit disorder," indicating the individual uniqueness and kaleidoscope of symptoms seen in AD/HD. Physicians must take time to determine what characterizes each child's case by carefully differentiating between symptoms presented. But is this really happening?

INAPPROPRIATE DIAGNOSIS

Results of a survey of pediatricians published recently in the *Archives of Pediatric and Adolescent Medicine*, revealed that doctors often spend less than an hour arriving at a diagnosis of AD/HD. Experts agree that this does not allow enough time for your child to be accurately diagnosed. The diagnosis of an attention deficit disorder is arrived at by compiling the child's history from several people, as we have seen, including the child. This, if done properly, obviously requires more than an hour. Therefore, if your child has been diagnosed quickly or by someone not qualified to do so, you should question the diagnosis and get another opinion.

"PUSHY" PARENTS

Doctors are not alone in rushing to give an AD/HD diagnosis. Amazingly, some parents push to have their child diagnosed and will "shop" among doctors to obtain the diagnosis they seek. They do this for two reasons, the primary one being to get the child on stimulant medication, which they view as beneficial for their child and others in the family. Some parents may even see medication as a convenient way to control unruly, not necessarily AD/HD, behavior, or the medication may seem like a foregone conclusion, having been suggested to parents by school authorities. Families on welfare in some states may qualify for additional benefits for each child diagnosed AD/HD, which also can be an incentive for parents to look for this diagnosis. Older children also have an incentive to be officially diagnosed as AD/HD because the disease has been officially designated an American disability. As such, this label earns a student extended time for completing standardized tests like the SAT, giving him a better chance to score well. It can also qualify a student for professional schools to which he might otherwise not be admitted.

MEDICATION ALONE IS NOT EFFECTIVE

The accurate diagnosis and treatment of AD/HD with medication have brought relief to thousands. Still, those who specialize in treating this condition agree that *use of stimulant medication alone is not the answer* . . . and a growing number of specialists reserve medication for those who do not respond well to other remedies. This group of physicians recognizes the importance of nutrition but, until now, have not had an easy program that their AD/HD patients can implement. My *30-Day Plan* was inspired in large part by encouragement from these professionals.

Even if you or your child is getting along well on medication, my *30-Day Plan* should be an essential part of the program. Learning how dietary change can turn around the life of any child or adult suffering from AD/HD is the message I hope to share with everyone reading this book.

HELPING YOUR AD/HD CHILD

The child with AD/HD, like the rest of us, is trying to figure out his place in the world and how to succeed within the family environment, at school, and with peers. He has to develop career goals, figure out how to meet them, and succeed in adult relationships. These children literally have a *different mind-set*, as we are discovering as we learn more about brain function. Therefore, during the developmental process, their self-esteem takes a battering as they struggle to be comfortable with who they are and how to take advantage of the considerable gifts they possess. The most important task you as a parent have is to help and encourage your child during this discovery process. If you are the partner of an adult with AD/HD, you have the same task, to help your partner achieve success by optimizing his or her natural abilities.

It is interesting to contemplate why we consider AD/HD the plague of the nineties—just as we are beginning to understand that attention deficits involve the brain's ability to focus on survival skills that have sustained humans for centuries. This mind-set has been with us all along— it's just that today the warrior/survivor types are trapped in an endless sea of "executive skills" to which they are ill suited. And those with brilliant creative minds are ridiculed for being "different" and not allowed to daydream. As we become increasingly sedentary and our dietary practices worsen, we will continue to have ever more individuals diagnosed AD/HD. The pathway we must follow to lessen the assault on the brain by this relatively new lifestyle pattern and improve self-esteem has to be nutrition.

I'm going to use a case history in the next chapter to show you how one family discovered their attention deficits and how they overcame the problem.

Understanding the Child with an Attention Deficit Disorder

I am going to introduce you to the composite sample of the Schaeffer family because they have struggled with the same symptoms of AD/HD in their son that you may be experiencing with your child or remember coping with as a youngster yourself. While Justin went undiagnosed for years, I will point out the clues that helped to determine he was suffering from AD/HD. The Schaeffers will reappear throughout the first two sections of *The ADD Nutrition Solution* as I discuss individual family members, their symptoms, and the significance of those symptoms.

THE NEW BABY—JUSTIN

There was something different about Justin from the very beginning. This second pregnancy had been much easier for his mother, Ann. She was not plagued with the nausea that had persisted throughout her first pregnancy. His birth went smoothly, and he was a healthy little boy. However, Justin had been restless in the womb and fussy from the time he came home from the hospital. His behavior was entirely different from that of his sister—who was eighteen months old. What Ann did not know was that the persistent nausea during her first pregnancy most likely contributed to Justin's behavior. It suggests that when she became pregnant with Justin, Ann was still low in several essential nutrients, such as fatty acids, minerals, and vitamins, which would cause a deficiency in Justin and add to his movement in the womb.

When Justin arrived home with Ann from the hospital he slept only two hours a day. Often he would doze after breast-feeding lightly, only to awaken again when his parents put him down. They would then pick him up and Ann would offer him more to eat, but many times all he wanted was to be held. Over time it seemed to his parents that Justin didn't get enough to eat and never slept. However, their pediatrician could not find any reason for his restlessness, and Justin was gaining weight normally and seemed to be doing just fine on breast milk. But, we know from AD/HD research that Justin's symptoms are classic for attention deficits. AD/HD children are often fussy babies and sleep poorly. Although they may gain weight, they are often not getting enough breast milk, which contains high levels of essential fatty acids needed for development of the brain, eyes, and heart.

The demands of the new baby infringed upon time Ann could spend with her daughter, Jennifer. Upon Justin's arrival, the little girl began whining and having temper tantrums to get her mother's attention. She deeply resented the intrusion of her little brother and demanded a place on her mother's lap whenever the infant was nursing. Worried about the impact upon her daughter, tired and drained from lack of sleep and increased physical demands of nursing, Ann felt waves of depression sweeping over her. Finally, after eight weeks of constant fatigue and strain from trying to meet the demands of both young children, Ann and her husband, Bill, decided to switch their little boy to infant formula.

The family situation was eased somewhat, because Ann was less tired. Jennifer didn't whine as much, although her temper tantrums continued and she still clung to her mother. Justin continued to wake frequently at night, and although it was less convenient to fix a bottle, at least Bill could share the responsibility for feeding him. Ann got a little extra sleep and no longer had the drain on her body imposed by breast-feeding. During the day, she had more time and patience to devote to her daughter. The little girl also seemed less threatened by bottle-feeding than she had by the close contact between her mom and the nursing infant. She enjoyed helping Ann hold the bottle for her baby brother and loved to entertain him with brightly colored toys. The family was finally on the way to adjusting to the newcomer. But while bottle-feeding helped this family greatly, the formula Justin was getting did not contain the fatty acids he required for very important brain, eye, and heart development. No formulas in the United States contain these nutrients, and because of this, Justin's AD/HD condition increased.

While much of his development seemed normal and on schedule, Justin was bothered by frequent ear infections from the age of six months onward. He sat unassisted at seven months, never crawled on all fours, but combat-crawled on his knees and elbows to get around until he took his first steps around the time he was one year old. Justin's language skills were confined to his own special lingo interspersed with an occasional word. This was attributed to his sister's readiness to translate for him.

At two, Justin developed a serious viral infection that required hospitalization. Following this episode, he was constantly bothered by a runny nose and fluid in his middle ear that put pressure on his eardrums. We know now that frequent ear and respiratory infections suggest an allergy to cow's milk products and that children low in fatty acids, such as Justin, are more prone to infections and have a tendency to urinate frequently, which Justin's parents noted as well. Other allergies are implicated as well by Justin's diet as a toddler. He was choosy about the foods he would eat, preferring milk, cheese, and hard-boiled or scrambled eggs. He liked fruit, mostly apples and grapes, and he loved spaghetti. The only vegetables he would eat were baby carrots and peas. He did not like meat or chicken of any kind, but he would eat turkey rolls and cocktail wieners. The only fish the family ate were fish sticks, which both children seemed to enjoy. Ann noted that Justin drank an unusual amount of fluids, mostly fruit juices. These foods, in general, contain many additives and allergy-provoking substances. As my discussion of AD/HD unfolds, you'll see just how these items can greatly exacerbate AD/HD.

Justin continued to be a demanding baby and was not good at entertaining himself. He was an extremely active little boy, running rather than walking every time he moved. When Justin did sit down to play, he sometimes had a hard time accomplishing activities that would seem to be within the capabilities of a child his age. His parents attributed his slowness in matching up simple shapes and colors to the constant interruptions from his older sister. Jennifer was quick to help out little brother when he faced a new problem, and her parents praised her for this. However, slowness in making associations between colors and shapes and not staying with the task until he mastered it suggests that Justin was demonstrating early learning difficulties and lack of small-muscle coordination.

Ann noted that it was hard to confine Justin. He was always trying to climb out of the shopping cart and didn't like his car seat or stroller, which made it difficult to take him anywhere. He liked other children but if he wasn't stopped, was likely to hit them on the head with whatever was at hand. On the playground, he would try to climb on the gym equipment but fell if he wasn't helped. This and other risk-taking behavior is commonly seen in AD/HD cases.

In spite of his difficulties, Justin had developed an engaging personality; he was very bright and a joy to his parents. He had just turned three, and his sister went off to kindergarten. Ann found he loved to fill his new time alone with video games, which is common with AD/HD children, who enjoy the fast-paced action and quickly learn to control character interaction and activity. Like most AD/HD boys, Justin preferred video games with action characters and would imitate on his big sister the quick defense techniques he saw his heroes use. Although his parents thought his play actions were typical little-boy behavior, Jennifer took the brunt of what were really his overly aggressive displays. In addition to video games, like the ones Jason loved, many AD/HD children will also watch videotapes for hours on end, and parents find welcome relief in playing favorite ones over and over again for their enjoyment.

At three and a half, his mother enrolled Justin in preschool, thinking he was bored and that contact with his peers and a learning environment would do him well. After two weeks, however, the preschool teacher called Ann and asked her to pick up Justin. The teacher complained that he refused to engage in normal school activities, was constantly pestering and disrupting the activities of others, and would not respond to any form of discipline. Ann didn't want to pull Justin out of school just yet and tried to talk to her son about his activities in school, hoping to change his responses. But, in the next few weeks, this behavior persisted until the school refused to keep Justin. Ann tried several other schools, with the same result. Usually Justin responded well to time out, but he needed time out so frequently, it was of little use in the long term. Even at this young age, Justin's lack of control over his impulsive aggressive and disruptive behaviors was becoming a problem.

In the meantime, Justin's behavior at home worsened. He would lash out at his parents when they attempted to correct him, or even if they tried to coax him to eat when he didn't want to. They had to keep him away from Jennifer because he now tormented her constantly. The normal discipline Justin's parents had once relied on didn't seem to work anymore. No matter what the outcome, once Justin embarked on a course of action, he was determined to follow it through. His parents worried that he would injure himself or someone else. They made sure anything hazardous was safely locked up. Justin's parents' fears were warranted: young children with AD/HD can seriously harm themselves or others because they have no understanding of the outcome of their behavior.

As for the family dynamic, crisis mode seemed to be the only one that operated anymore. Family outings became a nightmare because Justin would dart away from his parents at every opportunity and was very difficult to catch. Once they lost sight of him at the beach. They had just collected the lunch basket and gathered up a blanket, but when they turned to get Justin, he was gone. Several minutes of sheer panic followed while Ann and Bill frantically searched for their little boy. Terrified, they secured the help of a nearby ranger. While describing the child to the ranger, they spotted Justin walking close to the surf nearly two hundred yards away. The ranger's pickup got Justin's dad quickly to where his son was, just before he was about to disappear from sight behind a cliff.

Justin's parents thought that his poor response to instructions was perhaps the result of impaired hearing. They consulted their pediatrician when their son was four because they wondered if Justin's hearing had been damaged by the frequent ear infections he'd had as a toddler. The pediatrician referred the family to an ear, nose, and throat specialist who said that there was fluid in Justin's ears that could be hindering his hearing. He recommended that small tubes be surgically inserted into Justin's eardrum. After this procedure, the ear infections stopped and Justin's hearing improved—but his behavior continued to worsen.

Besides being extremely impulsive, Justin seemed unable to carry the simplest task to completion. He never seemed to have a clear concept of time and what he was supposed to be doing. Attempts to train him to pick up after himself were of no avail. He would start to help, become distracted, and drop what he was doing. It was often the family pets that were the source of distraction; Justin loved to chase them around in circles.

At five, Justin went to kindergarten. His teacher was an older woman who had taught kindergarten for years. She loved children dearly and gave them lots of hugs and other positive reinforcement for anything they did well. Her classroom was bright and cheery and she maintained a pleasant environment, although she enforced strict rules for behavior. She allowed her class members plenty of free movement during dance and gymnastics but insisted that the children sit still during the short periods of instruction. Each child was encouraged to explore his or her own style of learning, and there were lots of choices. Justin responded well to her training, and she kept him busy with a variety of activities. When he refused to comply or acted out, she took him quietly to the prep room for a time out. He loved to please her and was responsive to her one-on-one attention, as many AD/HD children are. At home, it was a different story. Justin continued to be a terror. It seemed he vented all his pent-up energy from the day on his family.

At six, Justin entered first grade and began to have trouble from the start. His parents found it difficult to get him organized and out of the house in the morning, and twice he refused to go to school at all. His schoolteacher was a young woman who had several years' experience in primary grades. She was not a particularly warm person but was a very dedicated teacher. She had a high success rate with achievement in her pupils, but Justin was a problem. He could not sit still, frequently leaving his desk to check out something that caught his attention. He liked to talk out regardless of whether it was his turn, and did so at the most inappropriate times. He did not follow directions and could not be trusted either to complete his tasks in school or bring them back after finishing them at home. When confronted with his misdeeds, Justin would deny any wrongdoing. Several times, he grabbed the workbook and threw it across the room or at his teacher in anger and frustration. On these occasions, the teacher noted that the little boy's motions seemed poorly coordinated. Although he enjoyed the company of the other children, Justin didn't like to participate in games, fell off the balance beam, and hated playing ball, indicating continued problems with coordination in both large and small muscles. AD/HD children are usually the last to be chosen for teams because they may be clumsy or lack ball-playing and other athletic skills.

Finally, Justin's teacher called a conference with his parents. At the conference, Bill noted that Justin's behavior reminded him of his own at that age and said he was just a "chip off the old block." This was a clue—really the first one—that pointed to the hereditary nature of Justin's condition. AD/HD does run in families.

After her discussion with Justin's parents, the teacher suggested the problem was AD/HD and that he be given a stimulant medication to settle him down. At first his parents refused, preferring to first try more involvement in Justin's class, to see if that would help. Justin's teacher continued to insist that he needed medication. Teachers are qualified to spot potential AD/HD problems, but they are *not* qualified to either suggest AD/HD or use of stimulant medication. Yet we find, as in this case, that they frequently do so. Despite the best efforts of the teacher and Justin's parents, after some more time he still could not write his name well—often reversing the letters—could not find the correct words to express himself verbally, and had made little progress in reading. As in Justin's case here, dyslexia or the inability to execute language skills often accompanies AD/HD and has also been strongly linked to fatty acid deficiency. As for math concepts, Justin seemed to grasp them when explained individually but was unable to complete pages of simple addition problems. This also coincides with the typical AD/HD child, where math concepts are often difficult and only get worse as he or she progresses into the abstract thinking required for multiplication and division.

Justin's parents finally decided, during the second half of first grade, to have their son tested for AD/HD. Their pediatrician referred them to a child psychiatrist, who gave Justin a thorough medical workup. A battery of tests was performed by trained observers, and Justin's parents were asked to answer numerous questions regarding their son's early behavior. His teacher completed a questionnaire describing his classroom behavior, and the school psychologist came in to observe and record his comments. The professional team agreed on a diagnosis of AD/HD. However, each individual on the team had a different opinion about the coexistence of developmental disorders and oppositional and defiant behavior in Justin. They suggested that Justin's parents begin immediate treatment with stimulant medication (Ritalin) to control his behavior. The team also suggested a program that included behavior modification and one-on-one tutoring for subjects in which Justin was behind. The diagnostic procedure was correct and the difference of opinion among members of the diagnostic team is common; each member brings his or her own interpretation of the child's behavior into the evaluation process. The team recommended a complete therapeutic program that included behavior modification, tutoring, family counseling, and careful selection of teachers and classes. Justin was not referred for special education because he was able to function within the regular classroom with the addition of remedial classes in language and math. The team did advise medication that in their estimation would improve Justin's ability to function in school and be more manageable at home. Not surprisingly, this team followed the traditional pattern of not recommending nutritional change as part of their program. My hope is that the easy-to-implement *30-Day Plan* I present here in *The ADD Nutrition Solution* will change the way AD/HD is treated by making dietary consideration and change a large part of a multipronged treatment of this disorder.

Attention Deficits–
A Brief History

AD/HD is a condition that has escalated in the 1990s, which makes us wonder if it has appeared out of the blue or if it's been around a long time and just been called something else. Actually, this condition has been known about for many years, but its causes, patient profiles, known symptoms, and names have evolved. Even the treatment currently used for AD/HD has been an approach used by some physicians for sixty years. Let's trace the evolution of AD/HD, because it helps explain the blossoming number of people who are struggling with this disability and its complexity.

AD/HD was first described in 1902 by George Still, M.D., in an address to the Royal College of Physicians in London, England. His pioneering research was later published in the prestigious British medical journal *Lancet*. Dr. Still described twenty children who were aggressive, defiant, resistant to discipline, excessively emotional, limited in their attention, overactive, and prone to accidents. We attribute the same behaviors today to AD/HD. The terms ADD and AD/HD weren't known at the time, so Dr. Still used terminology appropriate for the

Victorian age during which he made his observations. He described the boys as overly "passionate" and possessing little "inhibitory volition."

Dr. Still called his boys "Fidgety Phils" and we don't know much about their background, other than the symptoms Still described. The prevailing belief at the time was that children who behaved badly came either from homes of the underclass, who lacked adequate parenting skills, or from orphanages. In either case, the children were considered neglected, or disadvantaged, in that they had not been instructed in proper "moral fortitude."

IT'S NOT YOUR FAULT!

You may be thinking to yourself that nothing much has changed. As parents of AD/HD children, we are still accused of neglecting our children and not teaching them proper behavior. We have all been victims of "the look" that others give us when our unruly AD/HD child acts out. We must resist the tendency to think our child's condition is our fault—that somehow we failed as parents—as others would have us think.

Attention deficits do not discriminate between classes of people, either. Children coming from a less-advantaged background are not any more likely to have AD/HD than those from a privileged group. The disorder encompasses all social, economic, and intelligence levels. The greatest number of cases are, in fact, male children of well-educated parents with above-average incomes. Since we have now ruled out social class, lack of parental education, and neglect as causes of AD/HD, what about illness as a cause?

THE CONNECTION WITH SEVERE INFECTION

An epidemic of encephalitis hit the United States in 1917–1918. After the epidemic passed, many children who had survived infection displayed symptoms similar to those described by Dr. Still. Encephalitis is a bacterial or viral inflammation of the brain that can result in a variety of disorders. These include impaired attention, hyperactivity, and impulsivity. In 1918, they were thought to be post-encephalitic behavior disorders. Numerous scientific papers were published on the subject, establishing the idea that AD/HD occurred because of some major trauma or infection. The infection or trauma theory persisted for many years, and little was available in the way of treatment. Then a rather surprising thing happened.

THE FIRST USE OF STIMULANTS TO TREAT HYPERACTIVITY

In 1937, physicians at Bradley Hospital in Providence, Rhode Island, began treating hyperactive, "problem" children with a stimulant medication called Benzedrine. It's known today as Dexedrine (dextroamphetamine). The amazing thing about the discovery of Drs. Charles Bradley and Maurice Loffer, leaders of the Providence team, was that stimulants were effective in treating most hyperactive children. Why these doctors tried a stimulant on children who were already hyperactive seems odd. It continues to be paradoxical that stimulants can reduce hyperactivity.

Until the Providence team reported their discovery, little had been published in the scientific literature on the behaviors we now call AD/HD, and the idea persisted that hyperactivity resulted from some trauma or infection. Physicians noted that many of their patients suffered the post-encephalitis behavior disorders following rubella (German measles) infection, and in the years following, doctors began to look for some organic or biological basis for AD/HD.

THE NAMES HAVE CHANGED BUT THE
CONDITION REMAINS THE SAME

The terms *organic drivenness* and *restless syndrome* were popularized by the medical profession, and AD/HD-like symptoms continued to be thought of as resulting from some trauma to the body. However, during the three decades following the Providence discovery, the search to find an association between AD/HD behaviors and brain disorders, whether from chemical or physical abnormalities, resulted in a growing amount of research.

In the meantime, AD/HD continued to be thought the outcome of some shock to the brain; this idea persisted through the 1960s. As a result, the term for these behaviors was *minimal brain dysfunction* (MBD). Causes put forward for such lasting effects were birth trauma, head injury, rubella (German measles), or severe viral infection that occurred either during the early stages of pregnancy or in children under two years. Lead poisoning was also considered a possible factor, because it was known that lead can accumulate in the brain and cause learning disabilities.

A child labeled MBD had several strikes against him from the beginning, many of which were due to the fact that MBD was thought a mild form of mental retardation. This made it extremely difficult for these children to be fully accepted by peers and adapt to the mainstream. Consequently, their future outcomes were often bleak. Many adults recently diagnosed as AD/HD were labeled MBD as children.

Children labeled MBD who were not retarded but were actually AD/HD suffered from poor self-esteem—a condition that for many has persisted into adulthood. Unfortunately, mental retardation was the only psychiatric classification for MBD in the mid-1960s, and there was no provision for children with disabilities distinct from that harsh diagnosis. They were all grouped together under the same heading, whether they were learning disabled, developmentally delayed, or had AD/HD. Amazingly, these archaic attitudes persist in some people's understanding of AD/HD even today.

Many AD/HD children grow up feeling they are stupid, lazy, or crazy. Most know they have the capacity to excel, but they just can't seem to put all the pieces together to do so. We must be extremely careful to distinguish AD/HD from labels such as "retarded," otherwise we are grooming another generation for a nearly impossible transition into productive adulthood.

The AD/HD adults who have been struggling to succeed in spite of their self-doubt are relieved to find out that they have a real disability, and the diagnosis ends years of searching for what is wrong with them. Only some are successful with medication, but most are extremely relieved to find that they do well on my nutritional programs.

HYPERKINESIS—NEW TERMINOLOGY

Researchers in the 1970s began to question whether brain damage was the cause of AD/HD. *Hyperkinetic syndrome* was the term chosen to describe a distinct category of behavior that did not necessarily result from trauma. Hyperkinesis described children who seldom sat still, talked incessantly, acted out when in groups, loudly demanded their share of attention, and didn't pay attention or follow instructions. These are all characteristics of AD/HD, as defined today by the American Psychiatric Association. Hyperkinetic children were less likely to be considered retarded, but their parents found them extremely difficult, restless, easily agitated, and very active. This is the first time hyperactivity was established as a behavioral disorder, distinct from brain-damage-based disabilities. The door was now open for exploration into other causes of hyperactivity. One of the first to be proposed was diet.

DIET AND HYPERACTIVITY

Benjamin Feingold, M.D., a San Francisco pediatrician, was one of the first to advocate a dietary basis for hyperactivity. In the mid-1970s Dr. Feingold was an extremely outspoken advocate for reducing hyperactivity by eliminating some foods and additives commonly eaten by children. These foods included sugar, chocolate, food additives, and foods containing natural salicylates. His findings were challenged by other researchers doing studies funded in part by large food manufacturers. These manufacturers were unwilling to have the huge profits made from additive-laden foods reduced by Feingold's attacks.

Researchers since then have validated much of Feingold's work, although few have found the high percentages of improvement he reported when the food eliminations he advocated were made in diets of those who were hyperactive. Even investigators who adamantly maintain that diet doesn't affect AD/HD behavior admit that some children are helped by eliminating certain foods and dyes from their diets. I have gathered the most significant studies on the effects of dietary modification on AD/HD and have used them as the scientific basis for my *30-Day Plan*. I'll share more on these studies later.

The term *attention deficit disorder* evolved in the early 1980s to describe children who could not stay on task, were easily distracted, did not complete assignments, lost possessions, could not sequence events, and skipped from one task to another. The term *attention deficit/hyperactivity disorder* evolved in the mid-1980s to describe those who were constantly in motion, often left their classroom seats, talked incessantly, butted into conversations, didn't wait their turn in line, and liked to take risks.

The American Psychiatric Association officially recognized the disorders as psychiatric disturbances, and listed the first set of criteria for them in the *DSM III* in the late 1980s. During the decade between 1980 and 1990, thousands of new research studies were published, making AD/HD the most studied American childhood psychiatric disorder.

As the 1990s approached, Congress was motivated by the explosion of AD/HD cases and other mental disorders to draft a resolution declaring the 1990s "The Decade of the Brain." George Bush issued a presidential proclamation to that effect in July 1989, setting the course for increased research on all brain disorders including depression, schizophrenia, Alzheimer's, Parkinson's, and senile dementia, as well as AD/HD. As a result, we have seen an enormous expansion of research on brain disorders in the 1990s. This has led to major strides in the use of diagnostic tools such as brain imaging for all of the conditions I mention above.

Scans of the living brain responding to external stimuli have revealed what is going on chemically in those with AD/HD. I will summarize what we have learned with these new tools about brain function in AD/HD individuals in chapter 11.

The next thing you, as parents, need to know is how to tell if your child's behavior is not AD/HD but just normal little-boy or little-girl behavior. This is the subject of the next chapter.

Typical Little-Boy, Little-Girl Behavior or AD/HD?

There are staggering numbers of children who are being diagnosed as AD/HD, and there is widespread use of stimulant medication for 7 to 10 percent of school-age boys and a smaller percentage of girls. Why has the rate of AD/HD grown so fast through the nineties? Are we confusing AD/HD with typical boy behavior not considered unusual just a few years ago? Are we perhaps overdiagnosing this disorder and overprescribing medication to treat it?

Few people had heard of ADD or AD/HD before 1990, yet today it is rare to find someone who doesn't know of a relative or friend who has AD/HD. We need to explore why there has been such a tremendous surge in the numbers of children—80 percent of whom are male—being diagnosed with AD/HD. Here are some possible explanations:

- confusion over the difference between normal and AD/HD behavior, especially in boys
- increased recognition and reporting of AD/HD by teachers
- too little accommodation for the needs of children with a "different" learning style

- a rise in conditions that cause AD/HD, which include environmental, nutritional, social, family, and psychological trends
- increased recognition of adult AD/HD
- more frequent—oftentimes inappropriate—diagnosis of AD/HD by physicians
- public acceptance of the label "attention deficit disorder"
- commercially self-serving promotion of the use of stimulant medication
- a change in the medical standards used to justify the prescribing of stimulants
- AD/HD coverage by the American Disabilities Act of 1990, which confers special exemptions

WHY CHOOSE MEDICATION?

Let's revisit Justin's family to see how easy it is for parents to accept AD/HD diagnosis and opt for medication. Parents of children like Justin may be relieved to find that their child has an officially recognized, controllable medical condition, and they may find the use of stimulant medication an attractive solution. Justin was a difficult child from the beginning, and his aggressive, impulsive behavior continued to escalate as he advanced through the primary grades. He was extremely disruptive at school and at home. He made life miserable for all those around him.

Medication offered the possibility that Justin could be happier and more agreeable at home, more successful at school, and accepted by his peers. Justin's self-esteem had been taking a beating, and medication might have helped him improve academically and socially. It offered Justin and his parents a way to build a promising future for them all.

Parents shouldn't be blamed for choosing medication as an option, and many physicians prescribe stimulant medication as an effective way to end disruptive behavior. But does long-term use of medication alone guarantee a rosy future for the child, as has been suggested by its proponents? For many, medication does bring welcome relief, but used alone without other behavior modifying or nutritional treatment, it will never address the source of the problem. In Justin's case, even low-dose stimulant medication (10 mg per day) made him glassy-eyed and unresponsive. Ann and Bill decided to discontinue it after a week, opting instead to try nutrition, behavioral, and educational modification.

IS RITALIN THE ANSWER?

Stimulant medications such as Ritalin, which is most widely used for AD/HD, will *not* cure it, but the relief it can bring to a child and her family may lend an opportunity to consider other approaches. Professionals agree that Ritalin, or other medications, should never be the *only* course of treatment used. Yet some parents find it convenient to control their AD/HD child with medication and don't seek other remedies. AD/HD is a multifactoral disorder and therefore requires a combination of treatments to adequately address its source. Chapter 9 will demonstrate why Ritalin should not be the *primary* treatment choice, but used in conjunction with other remedies and then only in very difficult cases.

LITTLE-BOY BEHAVIOR

Let's go back to Justin and compare his behavior to that of normal little boys. What was it about Justin's behavior that contributed to his diagnosis? How could his parents be sure his behavior wasn't just typical of young boys? After all, his father had acted much the same way as a child, yet had adapted and survived well into adulthood. The pattern is familiar in that in most families, sons and their fathers are the ones likely to have been faced with AD/HD. Why is it that boys are ten times more likely to be diagnosed AD/HD than girls?

Anne Moir, Ph.D., a genetics researcher from Wiltshire, England, was quoted in an August 19, 1996, *Forbes* magazine article entitled "An Agreeable Affliction" that questioned the widespread use of Ritalin for attention deficits as saying: "There are some reasons for using it [Ritalin] with some kids, but I'm quite convinced little boys are getting put on it [Ritalin] because they're little boys." Like many other experts, Dr. Moir is convinced that normal little-boy behavior is being confused with AD/HD. If this is the case, it could help explain why the United States has far more diagnosed cases of AD/HD than any other country, and why we use five times more Ritalin than all other countries combined. Is there something in the environment here that is causing an epidemic of AD/HD? Are we less tolerant of certain types of behavior in the United States, or are both boys and girls being labeled with something other than AD/HD in other countries? Let's further explore the reasons why AD/HD is so common in the United States and why Ritalin usage is so widespread. I will start with the possibility that normal little-boy behavior is being confused with AD/HD.

BOYS AND GENDER-APPROPRIATE BEHAVIOR

Many parents don't know that little boys adopt gender-appropriate behavior at a much earlier age than little girls, and they mistake these behaviors for aggression. Remember how Justin at age three emulated the action heroes he saw in video games? Justin's behavior was unusual, however, in his repeated aggressive attacks on his sister. Justin frequently hit other children and at age two that did not necessarily signal a problem. However, at age three, Justin should have learned that repeated aggressive behavior directed at others is not appropriate. At two years old, children are implosive, self-centered, demanding, and always testing the limits. Boys can be particularly aggressive, but once past two, a child should begin curbing much of this behavior. Two-year-old behavior in a four- or five-year-old is not appropriate, yet Justin behaved the same at five as he did at two. What you remember about your childhood behavior or see in your child as inappropriate behavior as compared to peers should be the first area you explore when looking to a possible AD/HD diagnosis for yourself or your child.

EARLY PREFERENCES

Infants show little preference for male or female behavior, but by the time children have reached three or four years of age, they demonstrate decided preferences for "boy" or "girl" objects. Parents of both sexes note that both sons and daughters may enjoy the same kind of toy, but that they often show gender preferences for different versions of the toy. The construction toy LEGO, which is offered in either primary or pastel colors, is a perfect example. Girls prefer the pastel-colored version over the primary-colored set. I will follow the path taken by boys first, and then contrast it with little-girl behavior and what this means for those of both sexes who have AD/HD.

By the time little boys enter kindergarten, they have adopted patterns of behaviors accepted as "male." They posture and adopt the language and ways of bigger boys and men. Many, if not most, have been taught that boys do not cry or show other emotions; they must be tough and independent. They have learned that males should dominate and take control of whatever situation is at hand.

Some little boys adopt male behavior with greater ease than others. Older brothers may be good role models and can help younger ones establish appropriate male behavior. Little boys, in trying to assert male independence, find it difficult to separate themselves at a tender age from their mothers. For those who naturally have a sensitive disposition and don't have a tendency to be strongly independent, this can be a painful experience. These children may be uncomfortable and confused by the aggressive, dominating behavior thought appropriate for males, and some will respond with bed-wetting, stuttering, or stomachaches. Others will not socialize well or will not want to let mom out of their sight; some will respond with behavior that is aggressive, oppositional, defiant, and excessively loud. During play, boys are normally aggressive, rough, and noisy; however, by the time they approach first grade, boys should have learned to leave such behavior on the playground.

Parents, and perhaps some teachers, may be confused about what is normal little-boy behavior and what truly signals a problem child or one with AD/HD. Some little boys are severely punished because of their loud, boisterous behavior when they are just being little boys. Others are allowed to continue behavior that is no longer appropriate for their age, and many are heavily influenced by the violence and aggression rampant in our society, both in entertainment and in real life.

When do you decide if your child's behavior should be professionally evaluated? Judging behavior can be difficult, but you might ask yourself these questions:

1. To what degree does the behavior occur; is it extreme, even disabling?
2. Is the behavior appropriate to the child's age?
3. Is the behavior appropriate given the place it occurs (e.g., loud talking on the ballfield or playground is appropriate whereas the same volume is inappropriate in church)?
4. How long has the behavior persisted? More than six months?

If you are unsure of the answers to these questions, seek the help of a professional trained in the field such as a psychologist, psychiatrist, or social worker, or ask for a referral from your pediatrician. If you decide your child's behavior is just a little more boisterous than you would like, but not severe enough to warrant professional intervention, follow my guidelines for making appropriate dietary adjustments first. In any event, you must take the first step by deciding if your child is exhibiting normal, age-appropriate behavior, or if the behavior is most likely abnormal and a possible symptom of AD/HD.

How do Little Girls with AD/HD
Differ from Boys?—Jennifer's Story

Justin's sister Jennifer was eighteen months older than Justin and the product of a very difficult pregnancy and delivery. Despite indications that she may have been severely deprived of important nutrients during gestation, she was of average weight at birth and seemed healthy. But clues soon indicated she might be AD/HD, just like her brother. Jennifer was fed infant formula because her mother could not withstand the physical rigors of breast-feeding. The pediatrician switched Jennifer to a soy-based formula soon after her mother stopped breast-feeding, because she developed colic and constipation. Jennifer had milk allergies from the start, and she was then bottle-fed without adequate supplementation of the fatty acids essential for brain and nervous system development. Unlike Justin, Jennifer slept well and seemed happy and content. She sat by herself at six months, crawled on all fours at eight months, and walked at thirteen months. She took great interest in everything around her and loved to travel in the car or stroller.

Ann returned to work when Jennifer was six weeks old, and the infant was placed in the care of her grandmother, who lavished her with love and attention. At eighteen months, Jennifer's life changed dramatically with the arrival of her little brother. Jennifer's nervous and cranky reaction to her new baby brother was not unusual, but for her it may have been an indication of future problems. Jennifer did not adjust well to her brother's arrival. So as a result, Ann and Bill decided it was best for the family that Ann take a leave of absence from work to spend time with her two little babies.

Justin's constant demands caused Jennifer to begin vying for her share of attention and whining whenever she did not get her way. Frequent stays with her grandmother failed to pacify her. She began to have persistent temper tantrums, nightmares, and frequent bouts of bed-wetting. Jennifer seemed very anxious about her brother's welfare and wanted to entertain him constantly. If Justin fussed, Jennifer ran to his aid. She always tried to pick him up and comfort him.

At three, Jennifer was enrolled in preschool because she was imaginative, creative, and very bright, and her parents thought she needed a challenge. They also reasoned that it would be good for her to have the companionship of others her age. Jennifer enjoyed the school and often played well with others, but her teachers noted that she liked to go off by herself, and sometimes seemed lost in her own make-believe world. She had mastered dressing herself and loved to pick out her wardrobe for the day, being careful to coordinate hair ribbons and socks with the rest of her outfit. Ann helped her daughter make her selections before she went to bed at night, but in the morning Jennifer would want to change the complete outfit. Understandably, this caused considerable tension between Jennifer and her mother.

Jennifer frequently had colds and infections, requiring routine use of antibiotics. In addition, Jennifer constantly complained of headaches and stomachaches. Jennifer always had a runny nose and circles under her eyes even when she was well—chronic symptoms of youngsters with the allergies that I have found are one of the main causes of AD/HD.

At just under five, Jennifer headed off to kindergarten. She got along well with her teacher and enjoyed the fast-paced activities. Her kindergarten teacher, like the preschool teacher, noted that she liked to go off by herself for imaginary play. Jennifer worked hard to please her teacher, but the kindergarten schedule was often fatiguing, and she usually took a nap when she came home in the afternoon. Ann had difficulty waking her daughter for school some mornings, and she suspected the change-the-outfit routine was a technique to avoid going to school.

In first grade, Jennifer often daydreamed and seemed lost in her own world. Her teachers asked to have Jennifer's eyesight and hearing tested because she didn't seem to hear instructions. These were found to be normal, so other reasons for her behavior were sought.

In addition to general daydreaming, reading and math were especially difficult for Jennifer. She could not get started on math assignments even though her mastery of concepts was at grade level at the outset. She would squirm in her seat and tap her fingers when presented with simple problems that she should have been able to answer. In word-recognition tasks, Jennifer forgot words she had easily recognized previously. When her teacher tried to admonish her, Jennifer would smile her lovely engaging smile, making it very hard to correct her. But eventually she fell badly behind due to her struggle with abstract concepts, which many AD/HD children experience.

Jennifer's mother made a special effort to pick up unfinished assignments from her daughter so that she could work with Jennifer at home. This took tremendous patience for Ann, because Jennifer did not stay with her task unless Ann sat right at her side. If Jennifer made a mistake, and she often did, she got mad and either scribbled all over the page or crumpled it and threw it away. But it was clear to Ann after some time that the one-on-one approach was helping Jennifer improve her ability to learn.

At the end of first grade, Jennifer's teacher recommended remedial work over the summer. A good tutor was found, and Jennifer responded well to the continued one-on-one attention. Ann also kept her busy with swimming and camp when she was not being tutored. Jennifer seemed to be maturing, and her parents hoped that second grade would go more smoothly. While Jennifer continued to have headaches, they occurred much less frequently. Her emotional stress was lessened, but she was still experiencing tension and her allergies continued.

Second grade started off poorly. Jennifer's new teacher didn't appreciate her squirming and finger tapping. Once school started, the headaches and stomachaches occurred more frequently and Jennifer began to complain that the other girls didn't like her. Ann was very upset when a new Brownie troop was formed and Jennifer was not invited to join. Ann decided to enroll Jennifer in other activities, such as gymnastics and dance classes. Jennifer loved this, and the activities seemed to relieve some of her anxiety. Like Jennifer, many AD/HD children have problems with peer relationships and consequently have difficulty developing healthy self-esteem. As Ann did, parents should choose activities that their AD/HD child enjoys and is good at so that they can gain self-confidence. Daily physical exercise is extremely important for AD/HD children because it helps the brain compensate for chemical imbalances.

Increasingly frustrated over Jennifer's continued lack of progress in spite of all the efforts made, it was not long before Jennifer's teacher told her parents that either they put the child on AD/HD medication or she would have her removed from her class. When Ann and Bill complained to the principal, she backed up the teacher. They went to the school board, whose chair suggested that Jennifer be tested for AD/HD. Infuriated, Ann and Bill put Jennifer on the waiting list for a private school but had to endure the rest of second grade with the same teacher. By the end of the year, Jennifer was crying frequently, and her stomachaches increased. She became more and more impatient and began to receive failing grades.

Jennifer's parents were undecided about what to do. On the one hand, their daughter was very capable and had an engaging personality. Admittedly, she was difficult to keep on task, but did this really signify AD/HD, or was the school simply not accommodating her "different learning style"?

JENNIFER—GIFTED OR AD/HD?

The term *gifted* has no accepted definition, but is measured in part by an I.Q. above 130. A gifted child is described by psychologists as possessing great physical and psychological energy, one who sets extremely high standards for himself, enjoys problem solving, and easily becomes restless. The gifted are further characterized as independent thinkers, unusually absorbed or preoccupied with tasks and often unwilling to accept authority. These are traits also seen in many with AD/HD, and it can be easy to confuse an AD/HD and a gifted child. This can be extremely confusing to parents who are struggling to understand why their child is "different."

Children with exceptional abilities, whether gifted or AD/HD, seem to have overlapping behaviors, and both groups of children have a different mind-set. However, there is a big difference in performance between gifted individuals and those with AD/HD. While both groups have several projects going at the same time, *the gifted child will complete the tasks, while the AD/HD child will not.*

While both groups of children are drawn to begin different activities frequently, gifted children can control their work patterns to achieve a high degree of performance. They are driven by creative interest and self-motivation, while the AD/HD child has little self-motivation and needs constant reinforcement. Gifted children placed in special programs that allow more free expression will blossom. The AD/HD child, on the other hand, does best with structure and simple, clear-cut directions. Often the latter group excels at activities like computer learning, which rewards quickly, grabs attention, and is very structured.

Jennifer's case is an example of a child in conflict who will respond well to a multimodal approach to AD/HD. She is the perfect model of how family history (Dad with AD/HD, undetected food allergies, and nutritional deficits early in life) can affect learning ability and lead to a diagnosis of AD/HD. Part Two of my *30-Day Plan* will explore factors that can undermine brain function and why diet is important. I will demonstrate how we eventually *unlocked the child* hidden within Jennifer's small body. For now, let's take a look at research that has been done on behavioral differences between boys and girls with AD/HD.

BEHAVIORAL DIFFERENCES BETWEEN BOYS AND GIRLS

Most of the studies done on children with AD/HD have been done on males because eight out of ten AD/HD victims are male. However, there was an excellent study on girls published in the *Journal of the American Academy of Child and Adolescent Psychiatry* in March 1997. Larry Seidman, Ph.D., and colleagues from the Harvard Schools of Medicine and Public Health compared neurological test scores from forty-three AD/HD girls with thirty-six non-AD/HD girls. The girls ranged in age from six to seventeen years, providing a continuum of behavioral differences throughout the school years.

Not surprisingly, the study found that girls with AD/HD have impairments in attention and achievement, as well as a greater incidence of learning disabilities. They do not, however, show significant impairment in "executive skills" like organization, memory, creativity, and planning.

The same Harvard group led by Dr. Seidman had completed a similar study with AD/HD boys two years earlier, and therefore they could easily make comparisons between the performance of AD/HD boys and AD/HD girls. Overall, the girls had impairment in attention and achievement similar to the boys, but the *degree* of impairment was less. AD/HD girls fared nearly as well in executive skills as their normal counterparts, while AD/HD boys scored lower in these areas than peers deemed normal. If AD/HD girls have little impairment in organizational skills, creativity and planning, what behaviors do they struggle with?

Compared to non-AD/HD girls, adolescent AD/HD girls exhibit a larger number of eating disorders, greater anxiety, and double the rate of depression. The AD/HD girl has less chance of popularity and a greater likelihood of developing poor self-esteem. These girls are less aggressive and loud than boys, more likely to be withdrawn, with mood swings and temper tantrums. Many adolescent and teen AD/HD girls have hormone imbalances that can cause constant menstrual problems.

While AD/HD boys channel their excess energy outward as they mature, sometimes becoming increasingly aggressive and violent, most AD/HD girls tend to focus inward. As we will see in the next chapter, some older AD/HD girls go on to become extremely defiant and oppositional.

CLASSROOM MANAGEMENT—WHAT IS ACCEPTABLE?

Most boys are more physically active and have different learning styles from girls. Some teachers faced with "problem" children may believe that medication is the answer to classroom management. Many have referred problem children to school counselors, and others have even demanded that children be medicated. It is not acceptable for schools to refuse education to a child because his parents will not medicate him, yet this is a widespread practice. AD/HD is not a new disorder, but this rush to medicate children is.

We need to seek better understanding of different learning styles between boys and girls, especially those with AD/HD, and learn better ways to accommodate the differences in these children. We also need to understand the impact of diet on brain function and be more discriminating in what we feed our children. How do AD/HD children get along as they progress through adolescence and into adulthood? That's what we'll explore in the next chapter. The findings may surprise you.

The AD/HD Child Progresses into Adolescence and Adulthood

Two euphemisms often applied to an AD/HD child are "late bloomer" and "gifted underachiever." These terms imply that the child will outgrow the age-inappropriate behavior and poor school performance. For some AD/HD children that will happen, but is that what happened to you or what will happen to your child? Can you expect your son or daughter to outgrow this condition? What kind of adolescent and adult outcomes are possible and what should you as a parent seek to encourage and avoid?

I am going to discuss briefly several studies of possible adolescent outcomes of AD/HD; this condition can have serious consequences if not treated properly. My intention is not to alarm you, but instead to show you how nutrition is the common thread that runs through many behaviors and why you must use it now to beat AD/HD, ensuring the most promising outcome for your child.

Children identified as AD/HD in the early 1980s are now young adults, and many continue to have AD/HD symptoms. Indeed you may be one of these individuals. If you are, you have no doubt adopted a lifestyle that accommodates your abilities.

CHILD-TO-ADOLESCENT OUTCOME

Mariellen Fischer, Ph.D., Department of Neurology, Medical College of Wisconsin, Peter Ackerman, M.D., and James Satterfield, M.D., School of Medicine, Center for Health Sciences, UCLA, have led several research teams that looked for a link between a particular kind of AD/HD and subsequent juvenile delinquency.

Dr. Fischer's group did an extensive review of cases of AD/HD children to determine if symptoms continued as they grew older. Their study's objective was to find out what kind of symptoms persisted and how to design better interventions.

This team found that as AD/HD children progressed through life, they had more family conflicts, were more likely to be held back a grade, had lower academic achievement, and sadly, often failed to graduate from high school. Few had finished college. The AD/HD individuals also had a greater incidence of conduct problems, antisocial acts, substance use and abuse, emotional problems, and impaired social competence as they progressed into adolescence and young adulthood. These facts are very troubling to parents with an AD/HD child, but we must confront them to underscore the importance of early and effective treatment.

Dr. Fischer's team identified a subset of AD/HD children, who were markedly aggressive, as the most likely to have serious adolescent problems. She and her colleagues therefore defined *marked aggression* as the most reliable predictor of severe adolescent behaviors, including delinquency. Dr. Fischer found severe adolescent behaviors were reduced when the entire family, and parents in particular, were taught how to correct the style of family interaction that is detrimental to the markedly aggressive child. Family counseling was promoted, along with multimodal treatment for the child that included medication, behavior modification, education accommodation, and counseling. In other words, for the markedly aggressive AD/HD child, family interaction and dynamics make all the difference in the future outcome for the child.

Dr. Ackerman and his colleagues looked at the effects on AD/HD outcome when combined with learning disabilities, and the results of their study were reported in the *American Journal of Orthopsychiatry* in 1977. They found that learning disabilities (LD) complicate AD/HD, and if these are not addressed, there is a strong likelihood that the AD/HD teen will experience conflict with authority figures. Consequently, learning disabilities, like marked aggression, are another key predictor of future AD/HD outcome, and unfortunately, learning disabilities often go unrecognized in AD/HD children here in the United States. AD/HD has been a catchall term for many disabilities, but the complex nature of AD/HD and LD needs to be clearly defined, and this rarely happens. However, a change of focus can effect a more hopeful outcome for AD/HD children. In countries outside the United States, learning disabilities are the disorders identified and treated, rather than AD/HD.

A satisfactory explanation has never been made as to why these differences exist in the categorization of symptoms as AD/HD or LD. Many reasons have been proposed to account for why other countries have many fewer cases of AD/HD and why they identify learning disabilities more frequently than we do in the United States. Two interesting parallel studies comparing differences in teacher identification of AD/HD types were done in the United States and Germany. Teachers surveyed in the United States identified nearly twice the number of AD/HD students as either hyperactive/impulsive or combined types, whereas in Germany, fewer than half were identified as these types of AD/HD. Clearly there are differences within the educational systems of the two countries, and we suspect this is true for other countries as well, since none have the high incidence of AD/HD we do.

However, how we define AD/HD in the United States and distinguish it from LD is the product of not only our educational system but social, cultural, and family issues as well. Perhaps we really are producing more hyperactive and impulsive children in the United States. These issues will no doubt be debated for years to come. Let's move on to a discussion of how AD/HD symptom severity, family interaction, and socioeconomic status might affect the future outcome of children diagnosed with the condition.

Dr. Satterfield and his research team approached AD/HD childhood outcome from the opposite direction. They studied two hundred juvenile delinquent boys to determine how many had been diagnosed with AD/HD as children. Among the half that had, the scientists checked to see if socioeconomic level had any connection with the outcome. Surprisingly, they found that the majority of juvenile delinquent boys with AD/HD had come from an advantaged background. This information led to the next question, what was it about the boys' backgrounds that increased the incidence of AD/HD among them and why had so many of them wound up institutionalized? The significant factor in institutionalization turned out to be use of *stimulant medication alone, without accompanying therapies* such as behavior modification or family counseling. You may recall the emphasis I placed on multimodal treatment for AD/HD in chapter 4. The results of these investigations have emphasized the need for combination therapies in effective treatment of attention deficit disorders.

Some parents think medication alone will treat their child's AD/HD, when in fact it may do more harm than good. The medication may possibly divert attention away from treatment aimed at the disabilities associated with AD/HD. These include poor peer relationships, poor self-image, antisocial behavior, family conflicts, and learning disabilities.

While these studies may be alarming to you, it should be noted that the majority of AD/HD boys and girls do not have markedly aggressive behavior and, therefore, have a more positive prognosis than those studied in these samples. As to therapy, nutrition is the bottom line because it affects behavior, whether AD/HD or delinquency.

In the early eighties, a colleague of mine, Alexander Schauss, Ph.D., director of Biosocial Research in Tacoma, Washington, reviewed several trials that used nutrition to treat institutionalized juveniles and adults. The diets provided had been designed to minimize intake of sugar-laden foods and beverages while supplying more nutritious and balanced meals. The results were impressive in that behavioral infractions were reduced and the inmates were less apt to fly off the handle. Did a large proportion of these individuals have AD/HD as children? It was noted in several instances that some of them had been hyperactive, which was the term for AD/HD used at the time of their youth. So, while we don't know for sure if the subjects of those trials were AD/HD as children, it wouldn't be so big a jump to conclude that some were and that their behavior improved with a change in diet. What about the majority of children with AD/HD—how did they get along as teens?

AD/HD CHILDREN AS TEENS

Daniel J. Safer, M.D., and his research team at Johns Hopkins University School of Medicine addressed the issue of teenage behavior in those with AD/HD. They concluded that AD/HD teens continued to have problems with lack of attention, but were generally less aggressive and hyperactive than those younger in age with the same complex disorder. The AD/HD teens also had a track record of more school expulsions, suspensions, and a greater dropout rate than their non-AD/HD peers. This study further emphasizes the need for early treatment of AD/HD with a well-designed program.

THE AD/HD ADOLESCENT GROWS UP

The progression of AD/HD teens into adulthood has been the subject of several studies published in medical journals since the mid-1980s. One that included both males and females was a 1995 study done by Thomas Achenbach, Ph.D., and his team from the Department of Psychiatry at the University of Vermont. For their study, the researchers undertook the massive project of recruiting teenagers aged thirteen to nineteen from across the United States, all of whom had AD/HD according to the *DSM III* criteria used at the time. The team administered several tests to determine AD/HD symptom severity, existence of coexisting conditions, and overall learning ability.

Six years later, the same group of teenagers were retested as young adults, aged nineteen through twenty-six. As expected, AD/HD symptoms continued into young adulthood for both male and female participants. But a surprising result from the findings was a dramatic change in the characteristic symptoms of some females. As they got older, these female subjects were aggressive and defiant, whereas before adolescence they were not. Male subjects, on the other hand, retained the characteristics of their pre-adolescent behavior. If they were aggressive and defiant as adults, they had been the same as teenagers.

Other investigators have confirmed the observations of the Achenbach team, namely, that young women may have behavioral outcomes not predicted from their childhood AD/HD. While boys may tend to show less aggressive, defiant behavior as they grow up, girls may increase these behaviors.

Researchers found that young AD/HD women also exhibit a wider range of behaviors than men, and are more likely to be withdrawn, anxious, depressed, aggressive, and irresponsible. The investigators defined "irresponsible" behaviors as missing deadlines, frequent lateness for appointments, and disregard for the property and rights of others. Many of these adolescent girls had received past comments such as "acts too young for age," "can't concentrate," "is confused or impulsive," "has poor school (or job) performance," and "fails to finish things." In other words, a consistent pattern of impulsiveness, lack of responsibility, and underachievement followed the girls into adulthood.

IMPORTANCE OF EARLY DETECTION AND TREATMENT FOR AD/HD GIRLS

AD/HD girls have not been studied as often as boys, and yet we can see from these study results that the prognosis for females with AD/HD can be worse than it is for boys. Attention problems persisting into the teens appear to be linked to future defiant and irresponsible behavior in adult females, more than in males. Teenage girls often have poor eating habits, generated in large part by their fixation on the perfect figure, that tend to supply too few of the nutrients needed for them to beat AD/HD. Identifying AD/HD in girls while they are very young and designing appropriate behavior habits and diet are extremely important if they are to have a strong chance to overcome their attention deficit.

The developmental pathways between the sexes are different, and those in females have not been thoroughly studied or understood. Research on AD/HD intervention and prevention for females is badly needed, and the distinct characteristics of the female syndrome need to be recognized and treated more appropriately.

To summarize the progression of AD/HD in children, we can say that AD/HD boys with marked aggression continue to be aggressive as adolescents and are at greater risk for brushes with the law. AD/HD girls, on the other hand, need not be aggressive as children to be aggressive as teenagers, and they display a broader spectrum of behaviors over the years. We can also determine that both AD/HD boys and girls who have learning disabilities have a poorer outcome than those without them.

Establishing the links between AD/HD in childhood and its coexisting conditions is important in understanding future behavior and designing appropriate protocols for treatment. I must emphasize the need for treating AD/HD children, especially the aggressive subgroup, with a multifaceted approach. Ritalin or other medication alone is never going to provide the answer. I think we can safely draw this conclusion even from looking at the few tests that have been done that highlight such a determination.

For best results, it is important for you to integrate the nutritional aspect of treatment provided in my *30-Day Plan* into long-term management of your child's disorder. If you have an adolescent who is having problems, my program can help overcome their disturbing behavior as well. The *30-Day Plan* offers the best way to beat AD/HD for life and should be an integral part of any treatment program.

Let's take a look now at the adult disorder, how it differs from that of adolescents, and how adults can adapt to their disability.

ADULT OUTCOME

According to many reliable sources, including the National Institutes of Mental Health, 30 to 50 percent of AD/HD children become adults with the disorder. Several studies during the 1990s have focused on this disorder in adults of both sexes. It has become increasingly clear from the results of these studies that those who had another condition, such as a learning disability, coexisting with AD/HD as children continue to struggle with both conditions into adulthood. As you recall, we saw the same pattern in AD/HD adolescents.

AD/HD adults who were known to have AD/HD as children are also more likely to be male, divorced, separated, and of lower socioeconomic status as a result of less education. These conclusions, which were published in an article by Dr. Joseph Biederman in the *American Journal of Psychiatry*, do not adequately represent women, because adult males were more likely to have been the ones identified as ADD in childhood. More studies will have to be done with women as subjects in order to draw any similar kind of conclusion regarding female adults with AD/HD.

Now, what happens to coexisting conditions that were identified in AD/HD children, as they become adults? The most common coexisting disorders seen in adults with AD/HD are antisocial personality disorder, conduct disorder, oppositional defiant disorder, substance abuse, anxiety disorders, enuresis (inability to retain urine), stuttering, as well as speech and language disorders. Generally, the features of the adult disorder mirror those seen in children, and if there were no coexisting problems in the child, there are unlikely to be any in the adult.

Given the fact that so much more is now known about AD/HD, it is common for many parents of AD/HD children to find out about their own disability when their child is diagnosed. There is a strong tendency for attention deficits to run in families, which I will go into more deeply in chapter 7. I frequently work with families to help several members overcome AD/HD, and one of the outstanding virtues of the *30-Day Plan* is that it works for entire families. In following the same plan, adults are helped along with their children. These adults are relieved to put a name to the struggle they have often had with different aspects of learning and socializing and are delighted to find diet can help them, as well as their children, overcome this condition.

Male and female adults with AD/HD have different patterns of the disorder. This isn't surprising, considering the emergence of the diverse female AD/HD symptoms seen in adolescent girls. Women with AD/HD display a wide range of behaviors, not necessarily linked to what was seen in them during childhood. Men, on the other hand, tend to show the same behaviors as adults that they had as children.

A common problem for AD/HD adults of both genders is past school failure, resulting in insufficient education for job success. It is clear to researchers, and hopefully to adults with AD/HD, that these school failures do not occur from lack of intelligence. Salvatore Mannuzza, Ph.D., and colleagues from Long Island Jewish Medical Center, New York State

Psychiatric Institute, and Columbia University College of Physicians and Surgeons launched a study on men who had been diagnosed hyperactive as children. All of the men had normal or higher intelligence quotients. The symptoms of hyperactivity had decreased significantly between childhood and adulthood, but other coexisting behaviors continued. These included antisocial personality disorders (18 percent), drug or substance abuse (16 percent), and continuation of AD/HD symptoms (11 percent). These conditions, added to lack of education despite normal intelligence and the frustration brought on by that situation, would significantly impact one's ability to live a successful life.

An AD/HD adult study done by a team from the Neuropsychiatric Institute at the University of California, Los Angeles, found a similar set of symptoms. This team discovered that adults of both sexes with continuing AD/HD-residual type also contended with anxiety disorder (53 percent), alcohol abuse (34 percent), and drug abuse (25 percent). These findings are certainly grim, but the prognosis for adults with AD/HD isn't as bleak as it might seem.

Among the adults I counsel, many are very intelligent and talented, and the good news is that they have learned to accommodate their disability. Some, however, have been hampered by their lack of organization (mostly male), anxiety and inability to nurture others (mostly female), job instability, and inability to maintain relationships (both). Others have received medication to help them function, and they are relatively happy with their lives and accomplishments. However, some do not do well on medication and are desperate to find solutions for their problems. The nutrition plan I provide here offers the promise of long-term help for all these groups of adults.

IDENTIFYING ADULT AD/HD

Identification of AD/HD in adults is based primarily on a person's history of ADHD symptoms during childhood. Since AD/HD was not a recognized disorder prior to the 1980s, adults must look for clues in past teacher comments, in their own memories, and in interviews with their parents to determine if they suffer from an attention deficit. Consistent patterns of behavior mark the adult with AD/HD. They include:

job instability	relationship problems
authority problems	forgetfulness
poor self-esteem	physical or emotional pain
disorganization	mental fatigue

sleep disturbances

isolation

unwillingness to receive
   instruction or criticism

prone to auto accidents

difficulty with coworkers

restlessness/boredom

poor short-term memory

impulsiveness

procrastination

excess energy

nervousness

depression

tendency to overestimate
   ability to complete tasks

underachievement

We all experience some of these tendencies from time to time. Does that mean we have AD/HD? No. What truly marks the AD/HD adult is the *persistence of the disorder* from childhood. To be diagnosed as AD/HD, the disorder must occur consistently before the age of seven and cause impairment to career and relationships.

How Adults Adapt to Life with AD/HD

We humans have remarkable adaptive ability and desire to overcome whatever problems confront us. Most, but not all, adults with AD/HD have figured out how to work around their disability. To illustrate my point, I will present the cases of three adult men who have made adjustments to AD/HD, each in a different manner.

Bill lives in Tennessee and identified himself as having had AD/HD since childhood. He had learned to use his high physical energy and creative mind to build incredible landscape designs.

At the time I interviewed Bill, he was constructing a meandering streambed and waterfalls out of decorative rock and cement. The finished project looked like nature herself had fashioned it. The stream was stocked with fish, water seeped out between the rocks, and at several points cascaded into the stream. A wide variety of ferns and plants, some of them blooming, nestled among the rocks.

This man related how he had come to terms with his disability and used his different view of life to create beautiful and peaceful garden scenes. He had made the effort to find out who he was and discovered a profession that suited him and gave him the feeling of self-worth and accomplishment we all seek. Bill's attitude typifies the resiliency of many adults who have made life adjustments to accommodate their differences. Long-term success in living with adult AD/HD means learning to realistically assess strengths and build on them. It also means learning techniques to prevent failure. Bill learned to use his physical strength and boundless energy to his advantage. An AD/HD individual who works in an office might use detailed to-do lists, carefully checking off completed tasks and resisting the tendency to procrastinate, thus avoiding the anxiety caused by piled-up paperwork, for example.

I came across another interesting case when I was giving a lecture in Buffalo, New York, in May 1998. I met a man there, named Don, who had an AD/HD son. Don ran his own successful business, despite having AD/HD himself. Both Don, who was divorced from the boy's mother, and his son were taking a low dose of Ritalin. Like many parents, Don had discovered his own disability when his son was diagnosed. After years of struggling to keep his mind focused, Don had found that Ritalin cleared the mental fog and brought him instant relief. He described the feeling as "putting glasses on my brain." He was well aware of the numerous side effects of stimulant medication and did not want to rely on using it permanently, especially for his son. Don also knew that medications do not provide lasting relief and that the dosage frequently had to be increased periodically. He was determined to use nutrition to help his son avoid going through what he had and to avoid the long-term use of drugs for his condition, so they were going on my *30-Day Plan*.

Like many single parents I work with, Don could control his son's diet only part of the time, because he and his wife had equal custody of their son. The boy's mother did pretty much what she wanted and didn't pay much attention to her son's nutrition. Nevertheless, the boy was impressed with how much better he felt and acted when he watched what he ate. On his own, he limited the amount of junk food he ate. Ultimately, like Don's son, each child must take responsibility for his or her own dietary decisions.

The last case I'd like to share involves a man named Jeff whom I met while lecturing in Baltimore. Of the three men, he had experienced the most difficulty in accommodating his disability. He was so scattered that he had difficulty verbalizing his story. As a child, Jeff had always had difficulty sitting still and finishing his work. He had gotten poor grades because he could not read, write, or verbalize well, but had made it through college because he was determined to do so. His job experience had been frustrating because he could neither get organized nor bring projects in on time. This had led to several job changes over a period of eight years. Jeff had also suffered numerous problems with fellow employees and bosses.

Jeff's stable relationship with his wife was one of the bright spots in his life. His wife was a grade-school teacher experienced in handling children with AD/HD. It was she who had urged him to have his disability diagnosed. He had tried a number of medications including stimulants that had made him nauseated and antidepressants that had left him agitated. Jeff was desperate to find natural alternatives to drugs. He and his wife together had identified caffeine and sugar as substances that exacerbated his symptoms, and eliminating these items from Jeff's diet had helped. He had tried various herbal remedies and supplements with limited success. Finally, he got on my *30-Day Plan* and has made remarkable strides in the past months. Amazingly, he got some relief almost immediately, but it took several weeks before he was able to function normally.

As experts have learned more about the progression of AD/HD into adolescence and adulthood, the extreme importance of managing the symptoms in childhood has emerged. Each child will be different and require multiple approaches to his or her condition. Much more research needs to be done on AD/HD in girls, since this group has been overlooked. Successful treatment of AD/HD in childhood can save the next generation of adolescents from developing more serious problems. It can also save thousands of adults from untold misery in the future.

Now, let's move on to the causes of AD/HD.

PART II

What's Causing This Problem?

Nothing you do for children is ever wasted.
They seem not to notice us, hovering,
averting our eyes, and they seldom
offer thanks, but what we do
for them is never wasted.

—*Garrison Keillor*

CHAPTER 6

AD/HD and the Environment

In the 1960s Rachel Carson tried to warn us of the harm we were doing to our environment with pesticides in her book *Silent Spring*. Few listened then, but over time others proved her theories correct. However, in the almost forty years since Carson's ground-breaking conclusions, amazingly few studies have been done on the neurobehavioral effects of pesticides and other toxins on children. In comparison there is ample research to demonstrate the harmful effects of heavy metals (lead, mercury, cadmium, arsenic) on the fetus and young child. In a recent search of MEDLINE, a medical research database on the Internet, I found over three hundred studies related to infants and pesticides, but almost all of these explored poisoning and obvious visible physical complications such as cleft palate or miscarriage. Only two or three addressed the question of neurological problems, and those studies were inconclusive. But in spite of the lack of research, is it not reasonable to assume that substances that can cause visible damage to the fetus or child can cause less visible damage to the brain of the fetus or child?

EFFECTS OF PESTICIDES ON BRAIN FUNCTION

One of the few studies that have been done was reported in *Environmental Health Perspectives* in June 1998. Elizabeth Guillette, from the University of Arizona, headed a team that included scientists from the Technological Institute of Sonora, Mexico. They recruited thirty-three preschool children from a Mexican valley and seventeen more from the nearby foothills. Valley farmers apply pesticides forty-five times during each of two growing cycles, and pesticide sprays are routinely used around the house. Because they grow different crops, the residents of the foothills do not use pesticides either inside or outside their homes. The situation provided the perfect test and control groups.

Both groups of children were tested for overall stamina, gross and fine eye-hand coordination, memory, and drawing ability. The results showed that those from farming communities in the valley were significantly impaired as compared to the children from the foothills. David Carpenter, a neurotoxicologist from Albany, New York, who reviewed the study results, was dismayed by the findings because the children in the valley had been exposed to levels of pesticides equivalent to those found in many areas of the United States. He noted that although cognitively impaired, the children did not show any of the other known symptoms of pesticide poisoning.

IMPACT OF PESTICIDES ON CHILDREN'S BRAINS

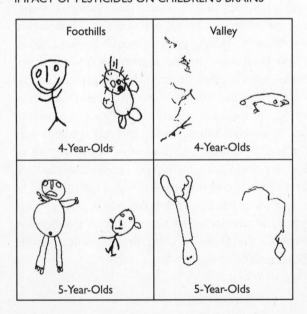

Foothills

Valley

4-Year-Olds

4-Year-Olds

5-Year-Olds

5-Year-Olds

These pictures of people were drawn by children from the foothills (no pesticides) and valley (pesticides) of the Yaqui Valley in Mexico. Note how being exposed to pesticides has reduced the children's small muscle coordination. J. Raloff, "Picturing Pesticides' Impact on Kids," *Science News* 153 (23) (June 6, 1998): 358.

The implications of this study for American children are clear. If children here are exposed to the same pesticide levels as the Mexican children, yet give no currently measurable sign that anything is wrong, might not pesticide poisoning be an underlying cause of their inability to sustain attention, learning problems, and hyperactivity? It really shouldn't come as any surprise that this landmark study clearly connects pesticide poisoning with cognitive impairment. Our surprise should be aimed at the fact that we have conducted no such tests as these until recently. We have been repeatedly warned by environmental groups that the level of pesticides normally ingested by children in the United States is great enough to cause significant neurobehavioral problems such as AD/HD. Now we simply have the proof to back it up.

The Environmental Working Group, a nonprofit research organization based in Washington, D.C., released a study in January 1998 with an alarming conclusion. The study declared that one million American children age five and under are exposed to unsafe levels of pesticide residues in fruits, vegetables, and commercial baby food. The group tested for pesticide residues in eighty thousand samples of food, and they detected average levels of organo-phosphates (commonly used to control agricultural pests) that were sufficient to cause long-term damage to children's brains and nervous systems.

Although the findings of this study were criticized by members of the food industry and the Department of Agriculture, the Environmental Protection Agency has since decided to review the study and make new recommendations on pesticide safety levels based on their findings. Young children are at greater risk for suffering brain impairments from pesticides or other environmental contaminants because their brains are developing at a rapid rate and don't have the protective elements in place that we adults do. As we get older, a selective filter called the blood brain barrier forms around our brain and protects it from most harmful substances. The barrier is not formed in children until after they are one year old.

It is for this reason that infants and the unborn are at greatest risk for many disorders affecting their brain development and immune systems. Fetuses are at the greatest risk, since toxins have a tendency to become concentrated in the mother and, while they leave her unharmed, to pass through the placenta into her unborn child. Lead, mercury, and chlorinated compounds are all poisons that play a role in altering brain structure in children both before and after birth. I will discuss in more detail how toxic metals disrupt brain function later in this chapter.

Where do these environmental contaminants come from? Pesticides get into children's brains from household sprays, food, and water. Pesticides are all around us, but there are steps we can take to protect ourselves. Let's begin by looking at food sources.

PESTICIDES IN FOOD

It literally boggles the mind to realize that each year, more than a *billion* pounds of pesticides are spread on fresh produce. We need to become more conscious of what is happening to our food supply, and take greater care to clean fresh fruits and vegetables before eating them. If the fruit or vegetable can be peeled (potatoes, carrots, apples, etc.), the problem is solved. For other foods (lettuce, spinach, cherries, etc.) just washing with water isn't sufficient.

WHAT YOU CAN DO: Many pesticides cling to produce and are not water soluble. To wash them away, use a good biodegradable cleaning agent such as "Lift," "Ecover," "Seventh Generation," or "Dr. Bronner's" and soak your vegetables and fruit. These safe, biodegradable cleaners will remove the pesticides and dirt, but they won't harm either you or the produce. Be sure not to mistake the type of product I am recommending with dish detergent! Carefully read the label—it will say whether the product is safe for food. Be sure to carefully rinse the soap off soaked vegetables and fruits before storing or eating them.

The other option you have is to buy organically grown produce. Organically raised products are always preferable to those that are not. With organic produce not only will you avoid pesticides but also fungicides, herbicides, and chemical fertilizers. You still have to thoroughly wash your fruit and veggies because even your backyard organic garden can be contaminated by pets or a passing raccoon. Many cities hold farmers' markets on a regular schedule and these can be a good source of fresh, locally grown produce. You are likely to find organic produce at these markets, but don't take the grower's word for it. Ask to see the grower's organic certification bearing his or her name and license number. Natural food stores and an increasing number of grocery stores are now carrying organic produce as well. Not only is organically grown produce safer for you and your family, but it often tastes better.

In your home, in the garden, and on pets use the most environmentally friendly pest control options. There are now many products to choose from that will help reduce or eliminate pests and not cause further harm to you family or surroundings.

WATERBORNE POLLUTANTS

Nitrates are a major waterborne pollutant. In large quantities they are a neurotoxin. The two most common sources of nitrates are commercial fertilizers and animal waste. We were made acutely aware of the effects of nitrate accumulation in our waterways in the fall of 1997. Great numbers of fish in Chesapeake Bay suddenly succumbed to an opportunistic bacterium, *Pfisteria piscicida*, that multiplied rapidly in the nitrate-rich waters. While the dead fish were a grisly and alarming sight, the bacteria didn't limit themselves to fish. Several cases of human illness involving fishermen and boaters who came in contact with the contaminated water were reported as well. Symptoms included acute neurologically based difficulties with memory and learning.

The source of the nitrates was traced to manure from large concentrations of chickens, hogs, and cattle raised on relatively small areas of land. So much manure had accumulated, that when heavy rains came, the holding basins overflowed and contaminated surface waters in streams and estuaries feeding into Chesapeake Bay. Nitrates from the manure accumulated in local waterways, and conditions were favorable for the unusual effects we saw in 1997. But what about nitrate accumulation in other parts of the country. Is it a problem?

The U.S. Geological Survey notes a large increase in the sales of nitrogen-based fertilizers over the past fifty years in this country. It reports that the greatest levels of nitrates in the soil occur in the upper Midwest, the East Coast, the Southeast, and isolated areas of the West. These are all agricultural areas with heavy use of commercial fertilizers. The result in these areas has been a contamination of ground water, most often drawn upon for drinking water. If you'll note the map on page 86 outlining the use of methylphenidate or Ritalin per state, you'll see that the areas of greatest concentration of fertilizer use and Ritalin prescriptions overlap.

WHAT YOU CAN DO: If you live in an area of high nitrate content and use a well for your water, have it tested regularly for nitrate content. Reduce your dietary consumption of nitrates and nitrites. Avoid lunch meats, bacon, ham, and hot dogs that have these chemicals added to them to retain color. Buy nitrate-free items. You will find lists of them in chapter 17 and appendix 2.

AIR AND MORE WATERBORNE PROBLEMS

There are a multitude of potentially harmful substances that we have introduced into our air and water supplies. Entire books concentrate on this issue alone, and so I am just going to mention a few that are thought to have the greatest impact on brain function and suggest how to reduce them.

Lead is a well-known neurotoxin. It was banned from gasoline a number of years ago because lead particles were being released into the environment from automobile exhaust emissions. In many states lead was replaced by methyl tertiary butyl ether, or MTBE. This additive oxygenates gasoline so that it burns cleaner. At first this move was applauded by many because it dramatically reduced levels of pollutants released into *air* from gasoline engines. However, what wasn't taken into account was that MTBE doesn't break down—it accumulates in *water*. Now we are having to rethink the use of MTBE because it has found its way into reservoirs and underground water sources that supply city residents with their drinking water. Jet skis and small boats with two-stroke motors that contribute the most to MTBE accumulation are being banned from reservoirs. Leaky underground gasoline storage tanks are being replaced

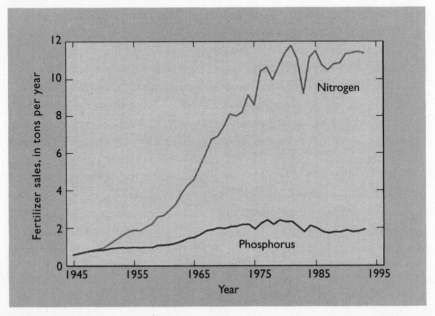

Fertilizer sales in the U.S. from 1945 to 1995 in tons per year. No. 113, U.S. Geological Survey Press, Government Printing Office, Washington, D.C., 1996.

with double-lined tanks. The only good thing about MTBE is that when it builds up in drinking water, you can smell and taste it, so you can avoid it!

While MTBE has been linked to numerous health problems, it isn't clear if AD/HD is one of them. However, animal studies involving MTBE strongly suggest that at high levels there is a risk of growth retardation and kidney problems in the unborn.

Chlorine is another substance that we must watch. Dangers to pregnant women from drinking chlorinated water have made the news in recent years. In February 1998 the *San Francisco Chronicle* reported that the California Department of Health Services had conducted a study that found pregnant women who drank five or more glasses of chlorinated water during their first trimester were twice as likely to have a miscarriage as those who drank less or drank bottled water. The trihalomethanes that formed in the water during the process of chlorination were blamed for the problem. The concentration had to be at least seventy-five micrograms per liter (75 mcg/l). This is high for most municipal water districts, but just to be safe, some water districts are changing to an ammoniated chlorine compound to avoid this problem.

WHAT YOU CAN DO: Check your local water source. If it's a municipal source, find out how they treat the water. If they are using more chemicals or additives (such as fluoride) than you are comfortable with, you can switch to bottled or filtered water for drinking. If you shop for an under-sink water filtration system, look for one that does not contain brass fittings. If you already have one installed, be sure to let the water that has been standing overnight clear the faucet before you fill your glass to avoid possible lead contamination.

The *San Francisco Chronicle* reported that a study conducted by a local environmental group found that home-filtered water may contain lead. The June 19, 1998, article reported that the lead levels detected in two water filtration systems exceeded the state level by sixty or seventy times. The problem was due to a design flaw that allowed water from under-sink filtration systems to stand in brass faucets. Filtered water has a higher acid content and can leach lead from brass fittings. However, if you let the water run before drinking, you should not be at risk for this particular problem.

WATERBORNE PARASITES

Numerous waterborne parasites can make us ill and adversely affect the brain. I am going to discuss the most prevalent one and how best to address the damage it poses. *Giardia lamblia* is familiar to hikers and campers who know the hazards of drinking untreated water from mountain streams. However, scientists warn that most *Giardia* infections occur much closer to home.

Summertime outbreaks of *Giardia* infection are the most common and are often due to improper maintenance of pool water and equipment. But even the best equipment can't guard against an infected child in diapers who pollutes the pool. If there is any reason to suspect the good health of a small child, keep him or her out of the pool. Day-care centers are the second most frequent source of infection as reported in *Time*, February 3, 1997. In addition, *Giardia* can cling to produce that has been watered with contaminated water and is one of the concerns of eating imported fruits and vegetables. However, if you follow my recommendations for washing your produce, you won't have a problem with *Giardia* or other waterborne infections.

Giardia and other parasitic infections can occur in young children and may be a source of hyperactivity, teeth grinding, bed-wetting, a dry cough that doesn't go away, itching in the rectal area, or headaches and dark circles under the eyes. Parasitic infections can mimic several symptoms of allergies, but unlike allergies, can cause diarrhea, fever, upset stomach, weight loss, and muscle pain when the infection first occurs.

WHAT YOU CAN DO: The good news is that parasitic infections can easily be detected through stool sample examination. If you or your child has AD/HD, I recommend that you rule out the possibility of parasite infection with a simple test. You will find resource listings for labs that conduct parasite testing in appendix 4.

ANTIBIOTIC USE AND INTERNAL ENVIRONMENT

Overuse of antibiotics has led to the well-known problem of some bacteria becoming immune to their effects. As we encounter the more pathogenic forms, we are finding fewer and fewer antibiotics that will kill them. Thus, physicians have lately become hesitant to prescribe antibiotics except for the most serious infections.

A bigger problem, and one that has gone largely unrecognized, is that antibiotics are not selective in the bacteria they kill. They kill all the bacteria they can find, including the friendly flora that live in our intestines. We need these flora because they produce some of the B vitamins we need to be healthy, they assist in digestion and absorption of water, and they produce metabolites that boost our immune systems. Diarrhea is a common effect of antibiotic use in children, and it occurs because all the flora have been destroyed by the medication. Amazingly, pediatricians still do not warn patients of this. Doctors should suggest that parents feed children yogurt with live acidophilus cultures whenever they are prescribed antibiotics.

WHAT YOU CAN DO: If your child has had repeated exposure to antibiotics, add acidophilus culture to his food, preferably the power shake I am recommending in chapter 11. You should also reduce your child's sugar intake, but you're going to do this anyway in my *30-Day Plan*. A good multiple vitamin and mineral is also included in the plan, to help restore your child's healthy immune function, feed his brain, and fight against nutrient depletion no matter what its cause.

If your child is prone to infections during a particular season, build up his resistance with herbs like *Echinacea*, *Astragalus*, and *Ligustrum* and increase his vitamin C intake. There are many good herbal combinations available for children and adults in natural food stores.

The total intake of chemicals from food, air, and water, our total environment, is what is harming us. Many environmentally related topics will be discussed in coming chapters. In the next section, we need to take a serious look at lead and its impact on the brain.

Do Heavy Metals Weigh Down the Brain?

Of course they do, but how big a problem is this? And, what can you do about it? Lead is the worst offender, and its devastating effects on cognitive function in children have been well documented. High lead levels have been recognized for a long time as causing hyperactivity, aggression, and even mental retardation in children. What has been discovered more recently is that even low levels of lead can also cause learning and behavioral problems.

In 1996, it was estimated that approximately three million children (12 percent) in the United States had lead blood levels of ten micrograms per deciliter (10 μg/dl) or higher. Concern over this lead toxicity has led the Centers for Disease Control to lower "safe" levels from 30 μg/dl of twenty years ago to 10 μg/dl today. Nutritional experts agree these levels are still too high and that no lead level is "safe." Given that, the fact that lead levels in our bodies are increasing with each generation is very disturbing. Especially since scientists comparing bone samples from people living today with those of ancient Peruvians (pre-Inca civilizations, prior to 500 B.C.) found that levels are now five hundred times higher than in our ancestors.

This lead accumulation can occur at a much higher rate in children than adults. Children are much more sensitive to lead levels than adults because of their smaller body size, and because more lead is stored in their brains, which are larger in proportion to their body size than the adult brain. In addition, the body's ability to eliminate lead is not well developed in children, so youngsters retain a greater proportion of lead ingested than adults do. Some children are exposed to excess levels of lead while they are still developing in the womb because lead readily crosses the placental barrier. Lead exposure during gestation is more likely to cause neurotoxic effects on the central nervous system (CNS) of the fetus than an older child's absorption of this metal because the unborn child is undergoing rapid growth and development of the brain and nervous system. It has also been found that levels of lead and other toxic metals are often higher in newborns if the mother is a smoker.

The chronic effects of high concentrations of lead in children are hyperactivity, temper tantrums, withdrawal, frequent crying for no apparent reason, fearfulness, loss of affection, listlessness, refusal to play, other emotional and behavioral problems, and learning disabilities. Physiological symptoms can include disturbance of body balance mechanisms, hearing problems, and reduced reaction times. Cognitive symptoms often include diminished intellectual development and poor reading and spelling ability.

Chronic exposure to lead in adults may cause anorexia, muscle discomfort, malaise, headache, constipation or diarrhea, metallic taste in the mouth, easy fatigue, poor muscle tone, insomnia, disturbing dreams, anxiety, restlessness, irritability, or abdominal pain.

Long-term effects of lead exposure are not fully understood but seem to result in deleterious effects on body organs, blood-cell synthesis, as well as nervous system and endocrine function. Lead displaces calcium and is stored primarily in bone. In other body tissues, lead displaces magnesium, zinc, manganese, copper, and iron, leading to possible metabolic enzyme function impairment.

Mental functions such as the ability to focus, hold one's attention, retain information, and demonstrate learning require calcium in the membranes of brain cells for information transfer between neurons. Lead reduces available calcium, so that messages become garbled and unclear. Energy to drive the communication between neurons depends on magnesium. Lead reduces the level of magnesium and other minerals that are needed for processing information, including manganese, copper, zinc, and iron.

AD/HD AND LEAD LEVELS IN CHILDREN

In 1966, Robert Tuthill, Ph.D., of the University of Massachusetts, Amherst, analyzed scalp hair specimens from 277 first-grade students in area public schools for lead content. Ninety-six percent of the students were Caucasian, and half were male. All were six and a half to seven and a half years of age, and their parents all had completed education beyond high school. This group of children came from an elite background, not the kind of environment we usually associate with lead toxicity.

In addition to the hair samples taken for lead testing, records were obtained from physicians, and questionnaires were completed by parents, school nurses, and teachers to help Dr. Tuthill assess AD/HD in this group. Allowance was made for teacher ratings for children who were medicated for AD/HD. The Abbreviated Boston Teacher Scale revealed that the higher the hair lead level, the lower the score. The children's hair lead levels varied from less than 1 ppm to 11.3 ppm (μg/g), and an even stronger relationship was observed between those with physician-diagnosed AD/HD and hair lead levels. The higher the lead level, the greater the number of diagnosed AD/HD behaviors.

LEAD SOURCES

The most common sources of lead are paint in older houses, some imported dishware, and more recently, imported vinyl miniblinds. You can obtain more information on lead sources from the Office of Lead Hazard Control in the Department of Housing and Urban Development. Fortunately, we have removed lead from gasoline, which was a significant source of contamination because in gas the lead particles were extremely small and entered the lungs where they were easily absorbed into our systems. However, lead doesn't break down in the environment, and so we continue to encounter it in soil and water. We tend to think that lead contamination is more likely to occur in heavily industrialized areas, but we must remember that lead particles are carried in air, rain, and groundwater, and can appear anywhere.

Lead paint is the most common source of lead contamination. Again, lead is no longer added to paint, but if you have an older house, and haven't painted it recently, lead could be a problem. Lead solder may still be used in canned foods, especially those that are imported. Lead glazes are still used for pottery in some locations, and water pipes may also contain lead.

Use of sludge for fertilizing crops can contribute significant levels of lead to the soil. The plants absorb it, as do the animals that eat the plants. By the time we humans consume the animals, lead levels have been concentrated one hundred times. Thankfully, the 1998 proposal by the U.S. Department of Agriculture to allow sludge as an approved "organic" fertilizer met with an overwhelming public outcry and was withdrawn.

OTHER DANGEROUS HEAVY METALS

Although lead is of the most concern as a cause of AD/HD, cadmium, mercury, and arsenic are also potential sources of contamination in ourselves and our children. Most of these heavy metals come from industrial sources. However, cadmium levels are known to be higher in cigarette smokers than in nonsmokers. By testing for lead and clearing it from the body, the other metals will be eliminated as well.

Toxic metals have accumulated in the environment, and they are not just on the surface. Analysis of tissue samples from people who inhaled ash-laden air after the eruption of Mount St. Helens, Washington, in the mid-eighties, showed lead levels four times higher than normal, cadmium twelve times, mercury three times, and nickel twenty times. Normal levels had been established for these individuals from previous clinical work. There is little we can do about airborne heavy metals, but we can check certain sources often found as contaminants at home.

COPPER PIPES—A SOURCE OF CONTAMINATION

I must mention that copper, although an essential mineral, can be toxically high in some children. Newer homes often have copper water pipes. It may be necessary to lower the copper levels because this metal interferes with zinc and iron utilization. I already mentioned possible lead accumulation from fittings in under-sink water filtration systems earlier in this chapter.

WHAT YOU CAN DO: Rule out lead toxicity by having a hair analysis done on you or your child. Hair is a very reliable screen for heavy metal burden, is easy to do, and is inexpensive. Labs that do this work are listed in the appendix. If heavy metals are a factor in your child's AD/HD, they can be chelated by vitamin C and will then be eliminated from the body. The *30-Day Plan* calls for supplementation of the essential minerals calcium, magnesium, zinc, copper, and iron, which are reduced by heavy metal burden, but if your child has elevated copper levels, it may be necessary to forego the copper supplement.

The Genetic Link: Born to Be Hyperactive?

Does AD/HD run in families? Yes. If there is one thing that all AD/HD specialists agree on, it's that the disorder has a genetic basis. That said, let's look at how this might affect your family.

ONE FAMILY'S HISTORY

There is compelling evidence that AD/HD runs in families. Take the Schaeffer family, for example. Justin and Jennifer were both diagnosed with AD/HD. Their father, Bill, had the disorder as a child, although as an adult he had adapted well. The only lingering symptom from his childhood was frequent migraine attacks. In chapter 8, I will explain how migraines relate to AD/HD.

Members of both Bill's and Ann's families had problems with AD/HD and related disorders. Bill's brother, Chuck, had a difficult time in school, with frequent expulsions. He was openly defiant, refused to abide by the rules, and resented having anyone tell him what to do. He had repeated two grades and barely graduated from high school.

Ann's family members tended toward depression. She had bouts of minor depression herself, and her brother, Kurt, had major depressive episodes. It seems that both sides of the family had a genetic tendency that was expressed as AD/HD in some members and as related problems in others. This may be typical of your family.

Let us investigate how the individual symptoms seen in the Schaeffer family might have evolved from a common genetic link.

THE AD/HD FAMILY

Justin and Jennifer differed in their AD/HD symptoms. Justin was more impulsive, defiant, and hyperactive, while Jennifer tended to be inattentive, anxious, and driven. Their mother, Ann, had occasional bouts with mild depression, and we'll look at that connection first.

DEPRESSION AND AD/HD: A FAMILY LINK?

You are probably thinking that any mother with two AD/HD children would have cause to be depressed. Others have thought the same thing. L. H. McCormick, M.D., looked for the answer to the question of which came first—AD/HD or depression—and reported his conclusions in *Family Medicine* in March 1995.

Dr. McCormick wanted to know if having a child with AD/HD increased the risk of depression in the child's mother. Not surprisingly, he found that it did. His fifty-nine subjects were biological mothers of AD/HD children who came from a small Midwest farming community. Twenty percent of the women in this group had minor depression, and 18 percent had major depression.

Comparing these figures to national averages for clinically diagnosed depression in outpatients, Dr. McCormick found that the women in his study had more minor episodes of depression (20 percent) as compared to the average (6 to 14 percent). They also had more major depressive episodes (18 percent) as compared to national averages (4 to 6 percent). Dr. McCormick used his findings to point out the need for screening the mothers of AD/HD children for depression.

The next question to emerge is whether these disorders are genetically linked or if mothers like those in Dr. McCormick's study are depressed simply as a result of their children's problems.

In September 1997 Stephen Faraone, Ph.D., and Joseph Beiderman, M.D., from the Department of Psychiatry, Harvard Medical School, presented their review of all the research that had been done to answer this question. They reported in the *Journal of Nervous and Mental Disease* that the body of evidence overwhelmingly supported a familial link between AD/HD and depression. "Depression in an AD/HD child should not be routinely dismissed as demoralization secondary to AD/HD, and depression in mothers of AD/HD children should not always be attributed to the stress of living with an AD/HD child." While one family member might be depressed, another might have AD/HD. Therefore, Ann's family history of depression was likely expressed in her children as AD/HD. What about the depression/AD/HD link on Bill's side of the family, especially in regard to his brother's anti-social behavior?

The Faraone and Biederman team found that AD/HD children who came from families with antisocial behavior had the greatest risk of depression combined with their AD/HD. Here's where home environment can make the difference in outcome for the AD/HD individual. In chapter 5 I discussed how subtypes of AD/HD strongly affect the adolescent and adult outcome for the AD/HD child. Now we see these subtypes emerging again as important factors in determining AD/HD outcome in families.

Another physician, David Comings, M.D., of City of Hope Medical Center in Duarte, California, has taken subtypes of AD/HD a step further by ranking severity of AD/HD first by what occurs with the attention deficit, and secondly, by how many family members have related disorders.

On the less severe end of the scale, he rated AD/HD coexisting with Tourette's (tic disorder) syndrome as less severe and AD/HD coexisting with conduct disorders as more severe. Antisocial behaviors in other family members were likely to result in more serious AD/HD occurring in children. The coexisting disorders were usually either conduct disorders or oppositional defiant disorders. The conduct disorders seen in Bill's brother, Chuck, were expressed in Justin as aggression. Is a genetic basis for AD/HD something new, or have doctors known about it for some time?

THE FIRST EVIDENCE FOR FAMILIAL AD/HD

J. L. Morrison and M. H. Stewart published the first study that showed a family tendency toward hyperactivity in 1971. They found that 20 percent of hyperactive children had a parent who was found in retrospect to be hyperactive. In the group of control children, only 5 percent had a hyperactive parent. This early study was followed by others in which mothers, fathers, siblings, and other biological relatives of AD/HD children were likely to have a history of childhood AD/HD.

Extending the investigation into second-degree relatives of AD/HD children, it was found that there is a stronger tendency for grandfathers rather than grandmothers of AD/HD children to have had the disorder. Similarly, uncles were more likely than aunts to have had AD/HD as a child. What is useful about these investigations is that they suggest a pattern of transmission for genetic potential that may be sex-linked. It has also been suggested that AD/HD in girls may be a more severe expression of the genetic root; we saw this concern expressed in chapter 5.

Just as we saw that as girls grew up, their behaviors could be more extreme than their male counterparts, so we see that female outcome is affected to a greater degree by related disorders in family members. Drs. Faraone and Biederman teamed up with colleagues in several medical centers to examine the occurrence of AD/HD in parents of girls with the disorder. They found the incidence of AD/HD in parents of girls the same as the rate for boys.

In the case of AD/HD girls, however, the parents had a higher incidence of antisocial disorders, major depression, and anxiety disorders. This would seem to support the idea that the disorder in girls is more serious. It is unknown whether the disorder is transmitted more frequently from the parent who is male or female. It appears from existing research that the various subgroups of AD/HD may be transferred by different pathways, but whether these are sex-linked is not clear.

HOME ENVIRONMENT OR GENETICS?

Environmental factors include medical problems, parental attitudes, classroom environment, peer relationships, and sibling response to an AD/HD child. To find out whether such environmental factors or genetic predisposition is a stronger influence on development of AD/HD, researchers have studied identical and fraternal twins.

In 53 percent of identical twins, if one had AD/HD, both did. Among different-sex twins both identical and fraternal, the percentage of both having AD/HD dropped to 33 percent.

What about children who are adopted? Does this make a difference in AD/HD outcome? The legal parents of adopted AD/HD children have been screened for childhood presence of the disorder. Only 2.1 percent of adoptive parents, as compared to 7.5 percent of biological parents, had AD/HD as children. If AD/HD occurs in adopted children, the influence of home environment is strongly suggested. However, this higher percentage of AD/HD occurrence in biological parents confirms a strong genetic link.

Dr. S. B. Campbell compared mother–child interactions between AD/HD children and non-AD/HD children. He found that mothers of hyperactive children provided more encouragement, impulse-control directions, and disapproval when compared to the mothers of the other group. Mothers do respond to their child's behavior and are taught special techniques to better manage behavior. "Time out" is one of the most effective tools in the management of an AD/HD child. Behavior modification is another tool whereby the child is commended for activities that would seem insignificant if performed by another child. If parents learn to look for activities that they can reward positively, the child will respond with less negative behavior. In doing so, parents are changing the *environment* of the child. This is where experts disagree over which is a greater determinant of AD/HD behavior, genetics or environment.

Numerous studies have shown a strong tendency for family patterns to be established in AD/HD children. This was especially true if one parent had antisocial or aggressive, angry behavior. In other words, there is a strong indication that some associated AD/HD behaviors are *learned*. Therefore, experts conclude that AD/HD is both genetic and environmental in origin.

AD/HD ADULTS AND THEIR CHILDREN: A PREDICTABLE OUTCOME?

The strong familial tendency of AD/HD might help predict future outcome of an AD/HD child. Joseph Biederman and colleagues investigated the histories of eighty-four adults with childhood-onset AD/HD. None of the children of this adult group had been diagnosed with the disorder. Of their children, 57 percent met the criteria for AD/HD, and 75 percent of these were treated for it. These percentages are much higher than those reported (20 percent) for the reverse situation in which parents are identified AD/HD based on existence of the condition in their children. Dr. Biederman's results support the validity of the adult diagnosis. The higher percentages of occurrence found in the children of AD/HD parents suggest that the adult syndrome has a stronger familial risk factor than the childhood form.

PRENATAL ENVIRONMENT AND AD/HD

Another factor that might account for the symptoms seen in Justin and Jennifer is Ann's prenatal history. In a 1995 study published in the *International Journal of Neuroscience*, researchers D. E. McIntosh, R. S. Mulkins, and R. S. Dean compared the prenatal histories of mothers of AD/HD children (74), ADD children (56), and normal children (135). All of the children were between the ages of six and thirteen. The research team found that the greater the number of a mother's medical conditions prior or during a pregnancy, the more likely a child of that pregnancy would be diagnosed with an attention deficit disorder. Additionally, if the mother experienced moderate emotional stress or smoked cigarettes during pregnancy, the child was more likely to be diagnosed with an attention deficit disorder.

Recall Ann's pregnancies. She was described as working and stressed throughout her pregnancy with Jennifer, whose delivery was complicated. Ann was depleted of nutrients going into her second pregnancy. Although her pregnancy with Justin was easier, Ann had problems during that pregnancy as well. All the female members of Ann's immediate family had a history of extreme nausea during pregnancy and very difficult first deliveries. With this family's history as an example, we get the first clues that nutrition may play a major role in the development of neurological disorders. A woman who is frequently nauseated throughout pregnancy has a hard time getting proper nutrition to support her growing fetus. We will examine this in greater detail later on.

CHAPTER 8

Food and Allergies That Contribute to AD/HD

DOES POOR DIET CAUSE AD/HD?

Why has AD/HD struck the United States population so incredibly hard? Could it be something in our diet that is contributing to the problem? Medical experts have traced the origin of many chronic diseases to unhealthy changes in our eating habits as a population over the past fifty years. We are repeatedly warned that cardiovascular disease, diabetes, arthritis, and cancer are all attributed to poor diet. Yet we have been slow to make the same association between diet and our fastest growing *chronic and lifelong disability*, AD/HD. We eat too much fat, sugar, and processed foods, and too few whole grains, fruits, and vegetables. I would like to share some information and the growing proof that these factors influence AD/HD occurrence.

The processed foods we love are loaded with over 2,800 additives that have been approved by the Food and Drug Administration as of June 1998. In addition, five million pounds of antibiotics and hormones are used each year to make animals grow faster and produce more milk. Common sense tells us that the overload of these items provided by the standard American diet cannot be good for us.

In the late 1980s the U.S. Department of Agriculture (USDA) became alarmed by the growing rates of obesity and other health problems common among our youth. They decided to investigate dietary practices among children and adolescents nationwide in order to account for this rise in diet-related disorders. Here is what they found.

How Do American Children Eat?

The USDA used a telephone survey between 1989 and 1991 to assess dietary practices among 3,300 children and adolescents between the ages of two and nineteen in the contiguous forty-eight states.

The results of the survey were processed and analyzed by Kathryn A. Muñoz, Ph.D., and colleagues from the Applied Research Branch of the National Cancer Institute. The results were published in the September 1997 issue of the journal *Pediatrics*.

The research team found that only 1 percent of the children and adolescents interviewed met *all* the national recommendations for daily servings of the five food groups. Sixteen percent of the youth did not meet *any* of the requirements. Even more shocking, nearly half the daily calories consumed by those surveyed came from fat and added sugar. I'm not surprised by these results; they confirm my own findings.

If our children and adolescents are not following the recommended dietary guidelines, what are they eating? I have asked this question repeatedly over the years, both in my nutritional practice and in consumer seminars I have given. Most of the audiences I address consist of people who were born in the last thirty to forty years. They have grown up with hydrogenated and processed foods, and may not have any idea that "real" food is different from these products they are used to. Additive-laden foods are so commonplace in today's American diet that many of us have no idea what unprocessed food is like.

For example, a debate rages about whether butter is better for you than margarine. The only healthy thing about margarine is its absence of cholesterol because it does not contain animal products, which are the only source of cholesterol. But margarine may contain trans fatty acids created by hydrogenation, artificial coloring, flavoring, emulsifiers, and preservatives. Saturated and trans fats impede the brain's ability to function. They are the worst thing an AD/HD individual can eat. I will explain more on this in chapter 11 and will show you how to scrutinize labels for unhealthy ingredients in chapter 16. Meanwhile, what other evidence do we have that poor diet can cause AD/HD?

FOOD SCIENCE AND AD/HD

Numerous scientists have investigated the action of food and additives on brain chemistry. Although there is widespread disagreement within the scientific community on the effects of diet on learning and behavior, there is a large body of evidence showing that diet plays a big role in AD/HD. What evidence from a clinical perspective do we have that these studies translate into real-life circumstances?

The coexistence of allergies and food sensitivities with behavioral problems has given scientists important clues about what is unbalanced or missing in the diets of AD/HD individuals. It has been known for some time that fatty acid deficiencies are common in allergic reactions. Symptoms of fatty acid deficiencies include dry, flaky, itchy red skin and scalp, eczema, raised bumps on the upper arms, hair loss, dry hair, brittle nails, frequent thirst, frequent urination, hormone imbalances, and acne. Many of these symptoms are present in children with AD/HD. Researchers began to look for fatty acid deficiencies in AD/HD children, resulting in one of the most important discoveries in overcoming AD/HD. Let's trace the clues that led to their discovery.

FATTY ACIDS AND AD/HD

Drs. I. Colquhoun and S. Bunday proposed in a 1981 issue of *Medical Hypothesis* that an essential fatty acid deficiency was a possible cause of AD/HD. They had noted that a large population of hyperactive children in West Sussex, England, were more thirsty than nonhyperactive children. Others among the hyperactive group had histories of allergy, including cases of eczema and asthma. Both conditions were known to be relieved by fatty acid supplementation, although other causes for these disorders were also recognized. Six years later, an investigation team led by Dr. E. A. Mitchell compared the fatty acid levels in blood serum between normal children and those with hyperactivity. (Remember that the term AD/HD was unknown at the time.) They found significant reduction in essential fatty acids, namely docosahexaenoic acid (DHA), dihomo-gamma-linolenic acid (DGLA) and arachidonic acid (AA), in the children with hyperactivity. Since then, there have been several well-conducted studies showing that not only do AD/HD individuals test low for essential fatty acids, but their symptoms can be *reversed* when supplements of DHA or, in some cases, also GLA, the direct precursor of DGLA, are provided. Bottle-fed infants, up to the age of two, should also be given AA, as they are unable to receive enough from dietary precursors to meet the demands of their rapidly developing brain, eyes, and nervous system.

There are some other foods that do not cause allergies, but have been suspected of contributing to AD/HD symptoms in sensitive individuals.

NATURAL SALICYLATES

Herbs and some foods contain natural salicylates, such as white willow bark, which has been used for centuries to relieve pain. In fact, white willow bark provided the salicylate Felix Hoffman used to make acetyl salicylic acid, or aspirin, in 1887. He worked for a dye company called Bayer, and his discovery launched the pharmaceutical industry. We are all familiar with the pain-relieving properties of aspirin, which is chemically synthesized acetyl salicylic acid. Aspirin works, in part, because salicylates cross the blood-brain barrier into the brain, where they affect the natural morphinelike compounds that block out pain and elevate mood. These compounds are known as endorphins and enkephalins. For individuals with salicylate sensitivity, the powerful effects of these substances, whether they are synthetic or from foods, on the brain produce adverse symptoms. If you or your child cannot tolerate aspirin, you could be intolerant to foods, herbs, or flavorings that contain natural salicylates. A test is currently being developed that can detect sensitivity to salicylates. You can get information on the availability of this simple urine test from the Feingold Association, which is listed in the appendixes.

Foods containing salicylates include tomatoes, apples, apricots, cherries, grapes, raisins, nectarines, oranges, peaches, plums, and almonds. Wintergreen, a member of the mint family, also contains salicylates. This is a popular flavor for toothpaste, mouthwashes, breath fresheners, chewing gum, and after-dinner mints. As you read this list, you are probably thinking to yourself how often you or your child eats these foods. Apple and grape are two of the most popular juices and natural flavorings children encounter. As you start reading labels, you will find that many natural sweeteners come from grapes. These foods are not *always* bad for AD/HD individuals, only for those who cannot tolerate salicylates.

FORGET THE WINE AND CHEESE

Red wine can raise blood histamine levels in sensitive individuals. Paradoxically, it also contains substances called OPCs that prevent histamine release. OPCs are oligometric proanthocyanidins, which are members of a large class of protective phenolic compounds we get from fruits and vegetables that help strengthen the walls of arteries, veins, and capillaries, including brain capillaries. The addition of sulfites as preservatives to red wine appears to tip the balance between histamine release and retention in blood cells toward greater histamine release. Consequently, histamine "back ups" and blood levels rise, causing discomforts such as headache, drowsiness, and mood swings in those sensitive to high histamine levels. To make matters worse, we often serve cheese, which contains tyramine, a sensitizing compound in some individuals, with wine because the flavors blend so nicely. This combination may be the ultimate allergy snack, guaranteed to trigger a response in some people!

Any of the factors I've discussed in the last chapters, including environment, toxic metal burden, a genetic tendency toward AD/HD, allergies, and diet can contribute to attention deficit. When we consider them together, they are the pieces that make up the puzzle of what causes AD/HD. Only by addressing all of them will we be successful in overcoming AD/HD.

IS AD/HD A SYMPTOM OF ALLERGIES?

Allergies frequently occur in those with AD/HD. Specialists I have interviewed estimate that between 75 percent and 80 percent of children with AD/HD have allergies, specific food sensitivities, or a combination of both. Paul Marshall, Ph.D., from the University of Minnesota, is one expert who strongly believes that there is a special relationship between allergies and AD/HD behaviors in at least some hyperactive children. Family members may not have symptoms of AD/HD, but they often have conditions that experts maintain are allergy related. Migraines, mood swings, irritable bowel disorder, arthritis, eczema, chronic respiratory problems, and asthma are all thought to be allergy based. As we have seen, both Justin and Jennifer had attention deficits, and several related disorders ran in their family, including migraines, depression, mood swings, temper tantrums, and digestive upsets.

Conventional medicine views these conditions as unrelated, and consequently each is treated according to its primary symptoms, rather than by the combined effects of all of them. Strong evidence is emerging, however, that there is a common source of these disorders. More and more evidence is leading doctors and patients to believe that AD/HD, migraines, depression, and arthritis should all be treated first with nutrition rather than drugs.

ALLERGIC RESPONSE TO FOODS

Allergies are the body's immune system response to foreign elements. We develop allergies to foods either because the food irritates the organs it comes into contact with and they respond negatively or because small particles of the food escape undigested into our circulation, where blood cells respond to them with uncomfortable effects.

The immune system responds to the foreign presence—whether it's detected on the surface layers of digestive organs or in the circulation—with a cascade of defensive responses intended to destroy it. Defensive tactics include activation of white blood cells, production of immune proteins, and chemical signals communicated between immune cells. Signs of the body's defensive effort are inflammation, tissue swelling, itching, burning, sneezing, and redness. These signs of allergic response can be verified by several tests.

The specific kind of white cells (eosinophils) that respond to allergies will be elevated in any blood sample that an examining doctor analyzes from a patient having an allergic reaction. Immune proteins that the body produces during an allergic attack will also be in these blood samples. The clinician can find out which of several kinds of response the patient's body has mounted by analyzing the relative ratios of immune proteins such as immunoglobulins E (IgE) and G (IgG) in his or her blood. Thanks to highly evolved methods of diagnosis, further testing can reveal exactly what caused the allergic reaction.

ALLERGIES AND FOOD ADDICTION

A clue to which foods you or your child might be allergic is something called the *addictive response*. "Must have" foods are often those to which you are allergic. The body can develop a response to a provoking food that results in a craving for that food. When the food is withdrawn, the individual may become quite ill during the first days following elimination of that food.

TREATING AD/HD WITH NUTRITION

Treating AD/HD with nutrition results in significant improvement in symptoms. Experts like James Braly, M.D., an allergy specialist, maintain that four out of five children with AD/HD are helped by removing "provoking foods" and additives from their diet. What are these "provoking foods" and how do they affect allergies and AD/HD? As we saw from Dr.

Paul Marshall's research, the prevalence of any form of allergy, including food allergies, is much higher in the AD/HD population than in the general population.

The list of common provoking foods isn't long, but it does include milk, eggs, wheat, corn, chocolate, and oranges, foods that are encountered daily in the typical American diet. Frequent consumption of these foods is one of the reasons we become *sensitized* to them.

ELIMINATION OF OFFENDING FOODS

The *30-Day Plan* begins with elimination of the most common provoking foods for one month. AD/HD symptoms will usually improve during this period. You can then reintroduce the foods that you have eliminated, one at a time, noting your or your child's responses. This will give you a good idea if food allergies are contributing to the AD/HD. I will give you detailed instructions on how to do this in chapter 15. Right now, let's see what it is in foods and inhalants that causes allergies.

Foreign proteins cause the greatest number of allergic reactions, whether they enter the body through the nose, skin, or digestive system. In the case of food allergies, insufficiently digested protein chains, called peptides, can escape into the bloodstream and attract the attention of scouting white blood cells. These white blood cells first alert the other players on the immune response team and then proceed to attack and destroy the foreign peptides.

Foods can also be *psychoactive*, meaning that they have a direct and powerful effect on the brain. Sugar causes a psychoactive response, for example, in many of those with AD/HD. I will devote more to sugar's effects in chapter 10. Psychoactive reactions do not cause an immune response. Instead, they cause the brain to change the way it operates. In the case of sugar, the brain may become either more active or go to sleep. *Specific food intolerance* or *specific food sensitivity* describes foods that affect brain function but do not necessarily cause a typical allergic immune response.

I have reviewed many papers on the relationship between reactions to food and AD/HD. Many of these have been published by Paul Marshall, Ph.D., the aforementioned expert on the relationship between food sensitivities and ADHD. Dr. Marshall has emphasized that AD/HD children are more likely to have specific food sensitivities rather than food allergies, although they may have allergies to other things in the environment.

In fact, many of those who treat the AD/HD individual with nutrition recognize that a classic allergic response is not necessarily the only way a food can affect behavior. Roger Katz, M.D., an allergy specialist from UCLA, states that about 50 percent of the AD/HD patient referrals he sees have true allergies. Numerous scientific papers on allergies and AD/HD have stressed that non-immune-response food sensitivities are common in those with AD/HD. These non-immune-response reactions to foods nevertheless have profound effects on physical and psychological well-being in those who experience them. These effects include toxic reactions to specific foods or food items, altered enzyme function in the brain, direct action on brain neurotransmitters, and histamine release. Histamine is one of the brain's chemical messengers known as neurotransmitters. Histamine is active in both the brain and the nervous system. In the brain, histamine is concentrated in the hippocampus, an area of the brain responsible for consolidating newly acquired information. This helps explain why individuals suffering from either food sensitivities or allergies, which both involve histamine release, often have trouble remembering recent events. I will discuss the effects of neurotransmitters on AD/HD in greater depth in chapter 12.

Reactions to foods will generally be most severe when an allergic response to something in the environment occurs at the same time. Allergists refer to this as *allergic overload.* Typically, the environmental allergy is to some kind of inhalant from the child's environment—like mold, dust, or animal dander. Household cleaners and sprays are common allergens, as we have seen in chapter 6. Suffice it to say, the nondrug approach to treatment of AD/HD includes the elimination of common inhalant allergens. Let's explore the foods that commonly cause problems for the AD/HD individual.

Dairy Products and Respiratory Infections

Physicians practicing nutrition find dairy a prime suspect for causing food allergies. Among them is Doris Rapp, M.D., a well-known Buffalo, New York, pediatric allergist. Dr. Rapp has composed a list of foods to which most allergic children are likely to respond. In her books *Is This Your Child?* and *Is This Your Child's World?* Dr. Rapp puts dairy products at the top of the list of offending foods. My own experience in working with AD/HD individuals bears this out.

Lendon Smith, M.D., is another specialist who looks for dairy allergies in his young patients. A Seattle pediatrician, Dr. Smith maintains that dairy products are the number-one enemy of the child who has suffered numerous upper respiratory and ear infections.

Amazingly, we don't seem to outgrow our taste for milk even though we are the only species of animal that drinks the milk of another species. Americans consume more dairy products than any other nationality. We are convinced we must feed ourselves and our children daily servings of milk and cheese products to provide adequate calcium. In other countries, vegetables supply sufficient calcium for children's growth. We have a problem with this in the United States because only one-third of our children and adolescents eat the suggested daily servings of vegetables. While everyone realizes calcium is required for bones and teeth, it is not widely known that calcium is also vital for brain function. A dietary supplement of calcium is included in the *30-Day Plan* so that you and your children don't decrease your calcium intake with your decrease in dairy products.

WHEAT INTOLERANCE

A person's sensitivity to wheat is actually to gluten, the protein found in it. Eliminating wheat from the diet is difficult because it is in most foods. When you start scrutinizing labels, you will be amazed how often wheat is listed in the ingredients. We encounter it in bread, in pasta, as a thickening agent, as a coating, and in breakfast cereals. Hardly a meal goes by without some wheat! The wheat that is used almost exclusively in foods today is a hybrid wheat that geneticists developed in order to maximize crop yields, storage, and baking qualities. This means that we are constantly ingesting a specific kind of wheat protein with the result that we become sensitized to it. Older, nonhybridized members of the wheat family such as spelt and quinoa are less likely to cause problems because we have not become sensitized to the different proteins contained in them. These are therefore approved in the *30-Day Plan*.

"Too much, too often" is the same problem we have with eggs, oranges, and peanuts. The all-American breakfast includes wheat pancakes, bacon (nitrates, salt, saturated fats), eggs, syrup (sugar/artificial flavors), and orange juice. No wonder our children are having a problem with these foods.

INHALANT ALLERGENS WORSEN THE PROBLEM

Allergies often follow a seasonal course, particularly if the allergic person is sensitive to pollen and grasses. Molds can be a problem any time of year, especially in high-humidity climates, and they bother most people prone to allergies, including those with AD/HD. Pet dander can also cause problems, as can dust, glues, and other common household substances.

Management of AD/HD and allergies requires elimination of as many sensitizing substances as possible. Why are such a high percentage of AD/HD sufferers sensitive to foods and inhalants? Scientists believe an important clue lies in the brain itself.

THE EFFECT OF ALLERGIES ON ATTENTION

There is much debate in the scientific community on the question whether the AD/HD victim responds adversely to some foods because of specific abnormalities in his brain or whether he develops these abnormalities because his brain is responding to allergic overload. What researchers have found regarding the effects of foods upon the brain is not only interesting, but important enough that I have devoted chapter 11 to a discussion of these findings. This research is the basis for my recommendations in the *30-Day Plan* on the best time of day to eat certain food groups. My plan takes into consideration what science has revealed about the effects of foods and additives on brain function, especially in those with AD/HD.

The allergic response releases histamine in the brain, just like it does in other places in the body. One of histamine's effects is to increase the escape of blood serum into the surrounding brain tissues from within the thousands of tiny capillaries that nourish the brain. Eventually, the brain becomes waterlogged, and memory and attention are dramatically decreased.

HIDDEN ALLERGIES AND AD/HD

Allergies that impede brain function but show little evidence elsewhere in the body were first termed *hidden allergies* by William Philpott, M.D., and Dwight Kalita, Ph.D., in 1984. The hidden allergic response is very subtle—no itching, sneezing, or other obvious signs—which makes it so hard to detect.

Alan Gaby, M.D., of John Bastyr University in Seattle, Washington, believes hidden food allergies cause a wide range of physical and mental conditions. He wrote that identification and avoidance of allergenic foods can relieve a number of common and difficult-to-treat medical problems, including AD/HD, in an article published in *Alternative Medical Review* in April 1998.

A medical speciality known as "environmental medicine" recognizes, among other things, hidden allergies and treats the patients by determining what is inside or outside their bodies that is making them ill. The environmental specialist looks at the same factors I have been discussing, including pesticide and heavy metal contamination, overuse of antibiotics, allergy, genetics, and diet. Among the symptoms most commonly reported in chemically sick patients is lack of mental function that may or may not be AD/HD.

Sherry Rogers, M.D., is one of the country's leading experts on environmental medicine and is a past president of the American College of Environmental Medicine. She explains in her book *Depression, Cured At Last* that brain allergies are often not suspected in AD/HD and other mental disorders because the brain cannot reveal what is wrong with it. Unlike other parts of the body, no swelling is evident, and no rashes are present. Dr. Rogers notes that "when the brain has symptoms, it cannot wheeze and cough, it cannot break out in hives. But it can present a depressive mood." She further explains that the symptoms of brain allergies include seizures, migraines, rage, schizophrenia, autism, obsessive compulsive disorder, panic attacks, volatility, learning disorders, attention deficit disorders, and violent mood swings. Note that these are some of the very things that run in families of those with AD/HD.

ALLERGIC HISTORY AND THE AD/HD CHILD

Symptoms of allergies are commonly seen on the skin as dry, itchy patches, rough bumpy areas on the face, upper arms, and legs, and dry hair. Other symptoms are eczema, chronic stuffy nose, nasal catarrh, sinus congestion, halitosis, headaches, wheezing, or asthma. Some children may have experienced frequent stomachaches, muscle aches that were dismissed as "growing pains," rashes, and reddened cheeks or ears. Many AD/HD children have a history of repeated infections and frequent colds that seem to hang on. Fatigue, indigestion, constipation, bedwetting, and nightmares are also common in allergic children.

Stephen Gislason, M.D., another environmental specialist, has described some additional telltale signs of allergy in children. The allergic child often has "allergic shiners," bluish-brownish discoloration around both eyes. The shiners may be accentuated by puffiness under the eyes, created by fluid retention that leaves the tissues "water logged." The same condition is often occurring in the brain as well, leaving the child unable to think clearly. In addition, the whites of the eyes in these children may appear pinkish or red from dilated blood vessels.

It is important for you to know that allergies may have gone unrecognized in you or your child for years. Sensitivity to foods can contribute symptoms that do not show up until hours after an offending food is eaten, making it difficult to identify the culprit. Parental observation is the key to identification of allergies in the AD/HD child. Therefore, completion of the checklists for family allergies in chapter 12 is very important to your success with the *30-Day Plan*. Other clues to AD/HD allergies include a craving for specific "feel-good" foods. These are favorite foods that are most frequently eaten by the allergic individual and that may or may not precipitate a change in behavior. We'll take a look at the role of allergies and food sensitivities and avoiding them as a preventative measure against AD/HD, but first let's explore the role of medication in the treatment of this disorder.

AD/HD Treatment Options

STIMULANT MEDICATION WORKS—OR DOES IT?

The decision about how to treat your child's AD/HD is one of the most difficult ones you will have to make. Parents agonize over whether to begin medication or to look for alternative treatment options. The issue is strongly emotional, and parents are sharply divided into two groups, those who favor medication and those who do not. Often the parents of a child will be on opposite sides of the issue, and relatives add to the confusion with their own opinions.

If you are an adult with AD/HD, the drug option may represent a less emotional decision for you, particularly if it is to be used short-term and with other treatment options, such as psychological therapy. But even in adult cases, couples take opposite sides on the use of medication. Often the non-AD/HD partner welcomes anything that will alleviate the difficulties that the condition causes in adult relationships, while the AD/HD victim resists changing behaviors with which he or she has grown comfortable over the years.

In this chapter, I will present both drug and nondrug approaches to the treatment of AD/HD and show you why it needn't be an either/or decision. Medication may offer practically instant relief for complex problems but does not address underlying causes nor is it effective in the long run. Nutrition is a treatment method that takes longer but offers lasting results. Many find that a combination of these is the answer to their particular situation.

Doctors regard AD/HD as a neuropsychological problem and routinely treat it with stimulant medications, notably methylphenidate (Ritalin). There is no question that Ritalin has been of immense benefit to many families because it provides a quick fix for a complex problem. However, we must keep in mind that it is effective only when used in combination with other dietary and behavioral treatments. Thomas Achenbach, Ph.D., and colleagues stated the issue clearly in an article published in the *Journal of the American Academy of Child and Adolescent Psychiatry* in May 1995. "An important question for physicians to consider is whether stimulant medication alone results in more harm than benefit to the child and his family, since it may convince the parents that the child is receiving adequate treatment and divert attention from the need for treatment aimed at other associated disabilities such as poor self-image, antisocial behavior, and learning disabilities." As you will recall from chapter 5, reliance on medication alone without other treatment options in childhood can result in a teenager who has extreme difficulties with authority figures.

Although stimulant medication appears to be relatively safe from a physical standpoint, and nonaddictive even when taken for long periods of time, what about psychological addiction, especially for a child taking it through grade and high school?

WHAT MESSAGE ARE WE SENDING OUR CHILDREN?

At the first sign of suboptimal performance, the medicated AD/HD child is often asked, "Did you take your pill today?" We all have an occasional bad-hair day, but for those with AD/HD a clear message is being sent. Personal responsibility for one's actions isn't as important as making sure to take one's medication. This establishes the belief that success depends on being medicated, and the more firmly planted this idea becomes, the greater the opportunity for abuse of stimulants.

Use of stimulants is not confined to treatment for AD/HD. The extremely broad definition of the syndrome can easily be applied to many disorders, whether they are neuropsychiatric disturbances or not. Adults have little difficulty getting prescriptions for stimulants in order to improve work performance and enhance mood. This presents a significant danger in that use of stimulants will be viewed as just another tool to guarantee more consistent results and increased output. In a bizarre turn of events, therapists even report cases of parents stealing their child's medication for their own cognitive enhancement.

THE PROZAC GENERATION

Many professionals have the attitude that stimulants should be used to control AD/HD in the same manner insulin is used to control diabetes, aspirin is used to control a headache, or even the use of glasses for controlling vision. There are glaring problems with this line of thinking.

First, AD/HD cannot be defined as a distinct disorder with a clear-cut set of symptoms. Second, stimulants are effective in only two-thirds to three-quarters of the cases. Third, as a result of AD/HD much of the stimulant-consuming population today is young children. Fourth, the disorder is linked in some unexplained manner to one sex, which raises serious questions about the way our society views male versus female behavior. Boys are naturally more fidgety than girls, and this alone may make them more AD/HD suspect. Fifth, Ritalin or other stimulants do nothing to cure or correct the problems that are causing the AD/HD. Finally, stimulants and antidepressants are not harmless drugs, but heavy-duty controlled substances. We should be concerned that we have grown to depend on Ritalin so much that there was a serious shortage of it in 1995.

WHERE HAS ALL THE RITALIN GONE?

Ritalin sales grew from 50 million doses in 1986 to 350 million in 1996, a seven-fold increase, according to the DEA. And Ritalin usage across the nation is uneven. Comparing total recorded sales of Ritalin with population by state, we find the greatest sales occurring in the Midwest, the South, and the North Atlantic states. There have been no studies that look into why Ritalin sales are much higher in some states than in others. It could be that AD/HD occurrence is higher in the states where more Ritalin is sold, but other factors, such as overprescription or abuse may be involved as well.

ABUSE: According to the DEA, Ritalin is the fastest growing drug of abuse on school grounds. In the years between 1990 and 1997, overall sales revenues for Ritalin increased 600 percent to about $450 million annually, a situation unique to the United States, which uses five times more Ritalin than the rest of the world combined.

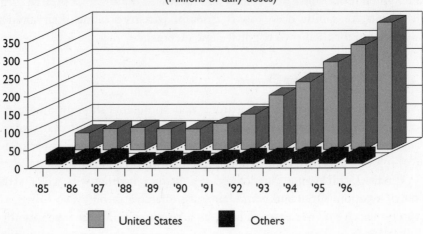

CONSUMPTION OF METHYLPHENIDATE
(Millions of daily doses)

Source: DEA report

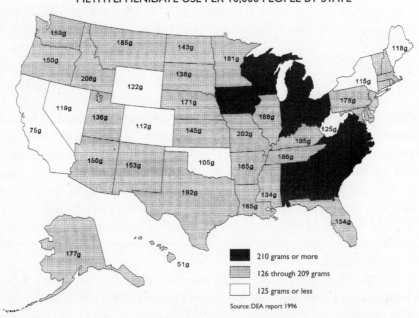

METHYLPHENIDATE USE PER 10,000 PEOPLE BY STATE

- 210 grams or more
- 126 through 209 grams
- 125 grams or less

Source: DEA report 1996

U.S. Average: 168 Grams
Annual Consumption for the Year 1996

ENTRANCE INTO UNIVERSITIES: Using AD/HD to gain entry into universities and professional schools has become so commonplace that according to the 1997 *Hastings Report* at least one major university has begun doing its own psychiatric evaluation of students for admission. Since a higher-court ruling has included AD/HD under the American Disabilities Act, students with this condition can gain extra time or a more favorable testing environment for the Scholastic Achievement Test (SAT).

OVERPRESCRIPTION: In a 1998 report issued by the American Medical Association, doctors admitted to "inappropriate" prescription of stimulants, including Ritalin. The AMA commission came to this conclusion after investigating twenty years of physicians diagnosing AD/HD and prescribing stimulants as primary treatment for AD/HD.

These days, the changing health-care system is likely to be a cause of further stimulant overprescription. After all, physicians are under pressure to spend as little time treating patients as possible. In this way, managed care dictates the most expedient and cost-effective way of quieting children. Unfortunately, until we make significant changes in health-care management, parents will be forced to do what you are doing by reading this book, that is, finding out how to help their children and themselves on their own.

HELP YOUR CHILD TAKE CONTROL!

Regardless of whether you have used medication for your child's or your own AD/HD, long-term success in living with this condition demands that you find additional ways to treat it. The statistics on the single-treatment approach to AD/HD show little long-term success. Despite use of stimulant medication in childhood, many adolescents continue to have major attention deficit symptoms as well as academic, emotional, or social problems without additional treatment methods. Yet we continue to use stimulants as the sole treatment for AD/HD without regard for behavioral therapy and educational accommodation.

Most children who use Ritalin must do so through adolescence. And it has drawbacks. This prescription drug sometimes causes insomnia, slowed growth, facial tics, depression (which must then be counteracted by prescription antidepressants such as Prozac), or liver damage. Many parents report that their children behave unnaturally when taking stimulants, have little zest for life, and appear to lack normal vigor and interest in what's going on around them.

In addition, no one knows how hazardous the constant use of stimulants may be over many years, because no long-term safety studies have been done. Many children take higher doses than needed, keeping them perpetually subdued. In some cases, children have discovered that they like the drug's effects and use Ritalin specifically to get high. Amazingly, Ritalin has even been promoted in the scientific literature as effective in cocaine withdrawal because it acts in much the same way as cocaine but has fewer side effects and does not cause a craving. We should use any drug this powerful with careful consideration.

It is truly a tragedy that so many youngsters and adults are regularly driven to take these potent and potentially hazardous prescription drugs when they may be unnecessary and the disorder they suffer from could be controlled in other more benign and safer ways. Changes in the diet and the addition of supplements can work just as well as Ritalin in controlling AD/HD, which has joined the growing list of American disorders that arise primarily from poor diet.

I am going to tell you now about two children for whom medication didn't work. The cases may seem extreme, but they do illustrate why you do not want to use medication alone without exploring dietary modification, supplements, and other treatments.

MEDICATION THAT DIDN'T WORK

One eight-year-old boy named Rich, whom I met during one of my counseling sessions, had a learning disorder rather than AD/HD. But a psychiatrist had misdiagnosed him and put him on 10 mg of Ritalin twice a day. It was a horrendous experience. Rich lost his appetite and became so listless he often fell asleep, even in the bathtub. When missing her son, Rich's mother would check his bed and find him taking a nap. This had never been Rich's habit before. As this abnormal behavior persisted, she decided to reduce his dosage of Ritalin to 5 mg per day, but that didn't seem to help. Rich continued to have headaches and finally became so agitated, he chewed all the skin from his fingertips until there was nothing but raw flesh! That last symptom occurred during the sixth month Rich was taking the medication.

When Rich's mother brought her son to me for advice after six months on Ritalin, she had already discontinued the medication one month previously. I started Rich on a change of diet and several dietary supplements that are the core of my *30-Day Plan*. Prior to beginning my program, Rich had been reading at about second-grade level, although he was in ninth grade. After three months on the diet and supplement program, Rich was reading at grade level. His math skills were still poor, but one-on-one tutoring by a college student was helping him to overcome his deficits. Rich had always been a good swimmer and decided to try out for the high school swim team. At last report, Rich, who is now fifteen, was doing well in school, had made new friends among his swimming buddies, and had taken charge of what he eats.

Another AD/HD diagnosed child, a little girl named Rebecca, came to me upon suffering detrimental effects of a 20 mg per day Ritalin prescription. After three months on this medication, Rebecca became quite depressed. As a result, her doctor added Wellbutrin, one of the "new" antidepressants that prevents excessive reuptake of serotonin from the synaptic cleft. The combination of these two drugs reduced the little girl's seizure threshold, a well-known side effect of both medications, and as a result she had a grand-mal seizure that lasted several minutes. In response, the physician advised antiseizure medication. When he added this final prescription, Rebecca's concerned mother gradually withdrew the Ritalin and Wellbutrin on her own initiative. The child's physician was so annoyed with the mother's decision that he refused to attend the girl and wouldn't return her mother's calls.

At this point I began to work with Rebecca's mother and had several conversations with Rebecca herself. Rebecca was very hard to work with because she was an extremely picky eater. But I made the limited dietary changes that she'd accept and relied primarily on supplements to treat her AD/HD. Her case shows that just using supplements is still very beneficial. The program just takes longer, three to six months, rather than thirty days, to work.

Occasionally, when she is having an unusually tough day, Rebecca's mother gives her one half of a 10-mg Adderall tablet. This newer stimulant medication is longer lasting and has fewer side effects than Ritalin, Dexedrine, and Cylert, the drugs most often prescribed for AD/HD. Like the other AD/HD cases, Rebecca's case reflects that a combination of several supplements is needed to get the best results. That is why my supplement program includes different classes of nutrients.

WHAT SHOULD I DO IF MY CHILD IS TAKING MEDICATION?

Read this book thoroughly, decide to try the program, and take this book to your doctor. Hopefully, he or she will find the information contained here helpful in weaning your child off medication, or at least in decreasing the amount needed. You may not be able to get your child to follow the entire dietary program, but even if your child is a picky eater, you can still reduce the additives in his or her diet enough to get beneficial results. In addition, the supplements I suggest correct existing imbalances, and every adult or child will improve to some degree if they are taken regularly.

Additionally, monitor your child's behavior carefully when you incorporate my dietary and supplement suggestions. Most parents report that the first thing they notice is that their child is less anxious, less agitated, calmer. As the supplements begin to help your child's body overcome the errors in brain function, you will probably find that he or she will need less medication. That's where your doctor will have to adjust your child's medications.

If you cannot get any cooperation from your doctor, refer to one of the agencies listed in appendix 4 for referrals to doctors in your area who work with nutrition. Now let's move on to the details of the *Thirty Day Plan*—dietary change for a lifetime!

CHAPTER 10

Treating AD/HD by Dietary Modification

WHY YOUR DOCTOR MAY SAY THAT DIET WON'T WORK

When your doctor says, "Diet does not affect attention deficit disorder," what he or she usually means is, "We do not know which one of these foods or additives will have adverse effects on *your* child." Most doctors are reluctant to try dietary therapy because it is time consuming and difficult to pinpoint exactly which foods and additives worsen your child's behavior. No single food is virtually *guaranteed* to worsen symptoms in most children with an attention deficit.

Nevertheless, it only takes a few days for there to be observable improvement in children's behavior when the *most likely provoking foods and additives are removed from their diet*. This makes diet the best place to start in overcoming AD/HD.

There can be as many as five hundred additives in any given food, according to a national press survey. Your child's system may be overwhelmed by the processed food he or she is eating. The cleaner you can make his or her diet from additives, artificial flavors and colors, processed sugars, and the other foods that often bring about allergic reactions, the fewer ADD-related problems he or she will likely have. My shopping guide, menu plans, and substitution charts will show you how to easily work around these symptom-provoking substances.

THE LINK BETWEEN DIET AND AD/HD: HISTORICAL PERSPECTIVE

The consumption of additives is extremely high in the United States. Many European countries have banned most of the additives we use. The Food and Drug Administration has estimated that the average child consumes between 150 mg and 300 mg of additives per day in processed foods, beverages, and candy. This level is three to four times the amount used in some clinical trials that had caused hyperactive behavior to worsen in children. I believe this is one of the primary reasons why we have such a high incidence of attention deficits and behavioral disorders in American youth. It is extremely important that you eliminate as many additives as possible from your child's and your own diet.

Dr. Benjamin Feingold was already widely known as an authority on controlling children's behavior with dietary intervention by the time he published his clinical findings in the 1975 book *Why Is Your Child Hyperactive?* Working with Kaiser Permanente Hospital, he developed the "Feingold Diet" (K-P Diet), which has been, and continues to be, enthusiastically embraced by millions of parents.

FINDING PROOF THAT DIET WORKS

Mixed results in treating AD/HD with diet have been reported in the scientific literature since the mid-seventies. The proponents of diet maintain that those who have declared diet is ineffective used flawed testing and research techniques in their studies. In the case of additives, several studies were conducted that either tested for only one additive or used amounts too small to adequately reflect amounts normally consumed by a child eating a standard diet. Bernard Rimland, Ph.D., director of the Autism Research Institute in San Diego, California, has also pointed out that none of the research teams who conducted these trials checked the use of cough syrups, children's vitamins, or other medications containing sugar and additives that might have skewed trial results.

AD/HD individuals who respond adversely to sugar might be sensitive either to the food source of the sugar or the chemical residues remaining in it from processing. Some researchers have reported that sugar derived from cane or beets appeared to cause fewer problems than that derived from corn. Other observers have proposed that those who react adversely to corn syrup but no other corn products might be sensitive to the chemical residues. Still other investigators found that the time of day the sugar was eaten and what other foods were eaten at the same time affected the symptoms.

After Dr. Feingold attracted widespread interest in his reported success in modifying behavior through dietary modification, several research teams in the 1970s jumped on his theories and sought to either duplicate or disprove his findings. Widespread disagreement resulted. Diet was a hot topic throughout the late 1970s and 1980s—and the debate continues today. As a general rule, scientific investigators are always critiquing the work of others and it is hard to find a consensus among them, especially for something with as many different variables as diet.

Testing for food effects isn't as simple as running trials for a new drug, for example, because there are multiple factors in diet that cause problems. *No single substance can reliably produce AD/HD symptoms in the majority of children, all of the time.* The major obstacle to agreement among the scientists was the lack of uniform testing methodologies. Two groups of investigators, each looking for the same effects to be produced from the same group of substances, could use different methods that would produce conflicting outcomes.

However, in spite of these challenges, today there are several well-conducted trials that have found results similar to Feingold's when *all additives and a few foods* are removed from the child's diet. Many of the best trials were conducted outside the United States, where children are classified as having a learning disability more often than having AD/HD. Those who do meet the accepted criteria for AD/HD are usually checked for food sensitivities immediately. A few of these studies are regarded by U.S. scientists as well designed and are often cited in the scientific literature. These include published clinical trials by Bonnie Kaplan and colleagues from Canada, Joseph Egger, M.D., and associates from Germany, Katherine and Kenneth Rowe from Australia, Jocelyn Burlton-Bennet from New Zealand, M. H. Schmidt and team from Germany, and C. M. Carter from England. These research teams have strongly linked sensitivity to certain foods and AD/HD. Some notable studies done in the United States by C. Keith Connors, Marvin Boris, and Francine Mandel have verified this link.

Reviews of the body of literature by numerous U.S. investigators have proven dietary modification can and does reduce AD/HD symptoms. Meanwhile, scientists today have accepted a protocol for conducting these trials, and we expect to see further confirmation of the role of diet in AD/HD.

A FLAVORING AGENT'S EFFECTS ON AD/HD

Monosodium glutamate (MSG) is an additive that enhances flavor. It is often used to prepare Asian dishes. MSG readily enters the brain, where it can affect the way brain cells communicate with one another. Approximately 30 percent of the people who regularly visit Asian restaurants have adverse reactions to MSG, causing "Chinese Restaurant Syndrome." As a result, many Asian restaurants now do not add MSG to their food, or will withhold it upon request.

MSG contains glutamine, the most highly concentrated excitatory messenger (neurotransmitter) in the brain. Dietary glutamate from MSG is readily picked up by the brain, especially when it is combined with sodium, as it is in MSG. Glutamate builds up in the brains of people who are sensitive to it, probably because they cannot process it efficiently. When glutamate builds up in the brain, it reduces the levels of other neurotransmitters. Ultimately, brain function becomes impaired.

The symptoms most commonly associated with MSG sensitivity include headaches, dizziness, blurred vision, nausea, weakness, thirst, flushing, burning, abdominal pain, cramps, vomiting, chills, depression, and dryness of mouth. The symptoms usually occur within thirty minutes of eating food containing MSG. Asian people are generally not sensitive to MSG for reasons that are not entirely clear.

A FOOD ADDITIVE'S EFFECTS ON AD/HD

Numerous studies have examined the link between food dyes, learning, and behavior. Most notable was a 1994 study published in the *Journal of Pediatrics* by Katherine and Kenneth Rowe from the Department of Pediatrics at the University of Melbourne, Australia. Theirs was a large study involving 200 hyperactive children who were put on a six-week diet that eliminated all synthetic food coloring. Based on the results of this and other studies, the most common symptoms noted with the ingestion of yellow dye #5 are behavioral changes such as increased hyperactivity, nervousness, anxiety, irritability, restlessness, and sleep disturbances. Of course, not all children will be affected by yellow dyes, but they may react to red dye #3 (erythrosine) or one of the other colors. In a 1980 study published in *Science*, authors J. M. Swanson and M. Kinsbourne reported that AD/HD children did poorly on learning tests given the day they received food dyes as compared to days when they had no food dyes. It also made a difference how much dye the children ate, which determined the severity of their symptoms. By comparison, children who did not have AD/HD were not affected by eating food dyes. Only by eliminating these from your child's diet will you know if they are at least partly to blame for his or her symptoms. All synthetic dyes and colorants are potential triggers.

In my *30-Day Plan*, I will teach you what to look for in the foods you purchase to eliminate as many of the synthetic colors as possible from your and your child's diet. You will become expert at reading labels before you buy any food. Colorants are listed many different ways. Complete lists of food and pharmaceutical colorants both natural and synthetic are given in appendix 1. Now, let's move on to how you are going to implement the *30-Day Plan* that eliminates these and other substances that can heighten AD/HD symptoms.

PART III

The Nutrition Solution Explained

Nutrition is life—you can have
plenty to eat and still have poor nutrition.
It's a matter of quality versus quantity.

—*Christiaan Barnard, M.D.*

How Food Affects the Brain

WHY SUGAR IS POISON FOR AD/HD

Many parents are convinced that sugar increases their child's hyperactivity and consequently they restrict its use. Other parents report just the opposite—their child is calmed down by eating sugar, in essence it provides "therapy" for the hyperactivity. Numerous studies have attempted to resolve the sugar issue, but none have found a clear connection between sugar and hyperactive behavior. What is the real story?

About twenty five-years ago, Dr. Benjamin Feingold warned that Americans eat too much sugar and that it could be a factor in hyperactivity. Since that time the idea has been repeatedly challenged by other investigators, but the truth is that nothing can be worse for people with AD/HD than eating sugar.

Investigators have been looking for *proof* that sugar will increase hyperactivity in *most* AD/HD children *most* of the time. They have failed to illustrate this point, because sugar's effects can be altered by whatever else the child has eaten either before or after the sugar test. They also failed to consider the broad range of response between individuals to the amount of sugar that can be eaten before it affects behavior. Even the time of day that was seldom taken into consideration. Finally, hyperactivity was selected as the only measurable effect of sugar when, in fact, sugar goes beyond influencing our energy level—it also has a profound effect on brain function.

New sophisticated brain-imaging tests, like positron emission tomography (PET) scans, have confirmed what Dr. Feingold and others have maintained for years: that hyperactivity is an adverse response to sugar. Now we know that it is not the only adverse effect.

PET SCANS REVEAL THE EVIDENCE

Such a study was conducted by N. L. Girardi, School of Medicine, Yale University, and colleagues and published in the *Journal of Pediatric Research* in October 1995. The study compared, by means of PET scans, the differences in response between AD/HD and non-AD/HD children fed a glucose-rich meal. Glucose is a simple sugar that the brain needs to function; we normally get glucose from dietary sugars and other carbohydrates. Seventeen children with AD/HD and eleven without it were given a glucose beverage before eating breakfast that contained approximately eight times the amount of sugar required by the brain in a single hour. That's about the amount of sugar you would consume if you ate a large sweet roll, a large glass of orange juice, and a cup of coffee with two rounded teaspoons of sugar. Both groups of children exhibited an expected jump in blood glucose levels within the first half hour.

HORMONAL CONTROL OF BLOOD SUGAR

Let me digress for a moment to explain briefly what this means.

The increase of blood glucose in these children was countered by a rapid rise in blood *insulin* levels, which was expected. Insulin's role is to move glucose from the circulating system into our cells, where it will be stored as a sugar complex called *glycogen*. Storage enables our cells to scoop up extra glucose and save it for later energy needs. Not all cells have this capacity for glycogen storage, however, and your brain cells are ones that do not. Your liver, muscles, and fatty tissues can all make glycogen, and they get the lion's share of glucose. The brain gets what little glucose it can immediately use, and even this meager amount can be severely restricted if insulin levels are high. Your body guards against the ensuing deficits in brain glucose in an interesting way, however.

Within three hours of eating a sugary meal, blood glucose levels drop back to normal or slightly below. This decrease in glucose triggers another important event that affects brain chemistry. The adrenal glands, two tiny organs on top of the kidneys, produce the "fight or flight" hormones *epinephrine* and *norepinephrine*. These hormones step up glucose entry into the brain, which offsets the effects of insulin.

In both groups of children, glucose and insulin levels dropped within three hours, as expected, but what Girardi and his colleagues found when they checked epinephrine and norepinephrine levels was startling. The AD/HD children showed an amazing 50 percent lower rise in these counterbalancing hormones as compared to their non-AD/HD counterparts. The AD/HD children *were less able to counteract the stressful effects on their brains* of the high sugar meal. Since norepinephrine is a neurotransmitter that increases alertness and the flow of information between brain cells, these findings were of major importance.

RESULTS OF GIRARDI'S TRIAL

A battery of tests measuring attention and learning ability were given to both groups of children a little more than three hours after their sugary meal. The AD/HD children scored significantly lower than the non-AD/HD children, which was not surprising and confirmed norepinephrine's role in offsetting insulin's slowing of brain function.

The investigators also noted that many of the AD/HD children had a *marked increase in physical activity* as their blood sugar levels plummeted. The researchers interpreted this as indicating they were using rapid movement, which increases levels of norepinephrine, *to jump start their brains*. Physical activity prompts the adrenal glands to pump out their hormones, which include norepinephrine.

Might hyperactivity then be considered the child's natural response to low levels of norepinephrine and glucose in the brain? I suspect, from my many years of working with AD/HD children and the evidence I have gathered from clinical trials, that this may in fact be the cause of *some* children's hyperactive behavior. If a child eats a sugary food on an empty stomach, the chances of it causing hyperactivity increase. Not all AD/HD children will react this way, but it explains why many do.

RISK TAKING: A SYMPTOM OF HYPERACTIVITY

I have interviewed many parents who report that their AD/HD child is a "risk taker," and this behavior has often been reported by others working in the field. This is another way a child can naturally elevate norepinephrine, and we see this behavior even in very young children. They climb all over the place and can seriously injure themselves trying to master skills for which they are ill equipped. The observations of Girardi and his associates help explain why risky behavior is considered by many experts to be a form of hyperactivity. What happens to AD/HD children as they mature? Do their bodies outgrow the inability to handle sugar properly?

To answer these questions a research team investigated how glucose utilization differs in the brains of teens with AD/HD as compared to those without the condition. Monique Ernst and colleagues, from the National Institute of Mental Health (NIMH) Laboratory of Cerebral Metabolism, tested 20 fourteen-year-old girls with AD/HD against 19 normal girls. Each girl was given a high-glucose drink and then tested for response to auditory signals.

AD/HD GIRLS AND BRAIN GLUCOSE

PET scans were again used to trace brain areas of high glucose concentration, indicating increased processing of information. The AD/HD girls had 15 percent lower glucose utilization over the entire cerebral cortex of the brain than did the girls without AD/HD.

Paradoxically, a similar test of boys revealed no differences in glucose metabolism between the two groups. This was a somewhat surprising finding, but may explain the tendency of some boys to outgrow hyperactivity, but not attention deficits. If, indeed, hyperactivity is an expression of the AD/HD brain's inability to get glucose into processing centers, the normal glucose metabolism found in these AD/HD boys suggests they may have "outgrown" one of the major causes of their childhood hyperactive behavior. Because they are attributed primarily to faulty neurotransmission, attention deficits can remain throughout life, although glucose metabolism plays a major role as well.

This study highlights the importance of gaining a better understanding of the differences in glucose metabolism between girls with AD/HD and those who do not have it, and between AD/HD girls and AD/HD boys. Teenage boys are much more expressive in their hyperactive behavior. They have been the subject of more research and are diagnosed with AD/HD four times more often than girls. The alarming thing is that girls seem less likely to outgrow impulsivity and hyperactivity. They express it differently, as short temper, fidgetiness, extreme procrastination, anxiety, and even depression. The future outcome of these conditions in girls might be better predicted if more studies on brain glucose metabolism were done. Do errors in sugar metabolism persist into adulthood?

BRAIN GLUCOSE METABOLISM IN AD/HD ADULTS

Alan Zametkin, M.D., another research psychiatrist from NIMH, published results of a trial in the *New England Journal of Medicine* in 1990
that answers this question. Dr. Zametkin found that adults with AD/HD
continue to metabolize glucose abnormally—at a rate 8 percent lower
than that of non-AD/HD adults. More importantly, glucose metabolism
was lowest in the prefrontal part of the brain, the section that regulates behavior, impulsivity, and attention—the very faculties impaired in
AD/HD. Although the frontal cortex was most affected, other specific
regions of the brain were also affected. Abnormal glucose metabolism in
the AD/HD brain appears to be a lifelong condition—at least in the
group tested by Dr. Zametkin. Clearly, this avenue of impaired brain
metabolism needs to be further investigated.

The adult men and women in Dr. Zametkin's study had a history of
hyperactivity as children, and each had at least one child with the condition. A strong case can be made for faulty glucose metabolism as the
genetic link that causes AD/HD to run in families. The findings in these
three studies are highly significant in that glucose is the brain's energy
source—vital for its functioning—and if the brain does not process glucose properly, energy deficits follow and communication between neurons becomes garbled. AD/HD individuals have described the feeling
inside their brains as having all the TV channels on at the same time with
the volume turned up. Stimulant medications "beam messages over the
gap" between neurons, thus bypassing blocked channels and easing the
static. While medication clarifies the signals between neurons, bringing
quick relief to many, it does nothing to improve the underlying problems,
one of which is faulty sugar metabolism.

We can overcome these errors in brain glucose metabolism by priming
the receptors to efficiently send and gather information. My *30-Day Plan*
addresses faulty glucose metabolism with better dietary management of
starchy and sugary foods and use of fatty acid supplements to repair neurons. Although sugar consumption by AD/HD individuals, regardless of
their age, must be avoided, it is especially important for AD/HD children. Here's why.

BRAIN NUTRIENT REQUIREMENTS IN CHILDREN

Amazingly, until the age of two, a small child's brain is using around
80 percent of the total calories he or she eats every day. By the time the
child goes to school, his brain is utilizing up to 50 percent of his caloric

intake. In addition, the greater size of the child's brain in proportion to the rest of the body demands a different ratio of protein to carbohydrate in the diet. We can apply this information to all our children, but especially those with AD/HD. What is glucose, and why is it so important to the brain?

Glucose is a simple sugar produced when we digest carbohydrates. Every cell in your body uses glucose to provide energy for cellular processes such as absorbing nutrients, getting rid of wastes, processing information, making proteins, and reproducing and repairing itself. Enzymes within the cell split the glucose molecule into smaller pieces. Energy that had been keeping the molecule intact is released and transferred to tiny storage units called ATP (adenosine triphosphate). All cells make ATP and use it as an "energy bank" upon which they can draw at any time.

Cells band together in functional groups called tissues to produce the products we need to live. For example, groups of cells making up respiratory membranes produce mucus that traps air so that we can breathe and that holds dust and other particles until they can be discharged. Other tissues like those in the pancreas produce the hormone insulin that regulates sugar metabolism in your entire body. Neurons, or brain cells, carry on many of the same activities as other cells, but unlike others, neurons churn out information twenty-four hours a day, every day of your life. Glucose is the only fuel your brain can use for this activity, and the demand for it is great. While other body cells can convert fats and proteins into glucose when extra fuel is needed, the brain cannot. Any disruption in the utilization or distribution of glucose in the brain—the control center of the body—will ultimately affect all body systems.

As we have seen, those with AD/HD appear to have a disruption in glucose metabolism in the frontal region of the brain. How, then, does eating sugar, the source of glucose, cause such a problem for those with AD/HD?

HOW SUGAR SABOTAGES BRAIN FUNCTION

Sugar can provide the necessary glucose to increase brain efficiency, and many of those with AD/HD do crave sugar. Yet, *eating sugar actually lowers brain glucose*, rather than raising it as might be expected. That's because our bodies still haven't adapted to a high consumption of refined carbohydrates like sugar. Only during the past two or three hundred years have we eaten sugar or sugary foods, yet today many forms of sugar have found their way into most of the processed foods we eat.

Over the course of human existence glucose has been provided by the slow release of sugar from complex carbohydrates, and this delayed insulin response. Our bodies are well adapted to handling a slower and more controlled release of glucose. Consequently, the body interprets a rapid rise in blood glucose from eating sugary foods as stressful and potentially life threatening. Let's look at what occurs.

When sugar enters our circulation after a meal high in carbohydrates, it triggers an output of the pancreatic hormone insulin into the bloodstream. Insulin insures that glucose gets into all cells and out of the bloodstream. The liver processes glucose and prepares it for storage. Some glucose from a meal will enter muscle tissues that also store it. Remember that glucose is a fuel, and the body provides it first to the largest soft tissues. If we engage in physical activities that demand muscular action, we need a backup in case of energy depletion, and our liver provides this.

Everything we eat and drink passes through the liver, which determines how each substance should be processed, even if it is harmful and should be destroyed. As a result of this process, the brain receives glucose that is released by the liver, but how much it gets depends on the amount of protein that is eaten along with the carbohydrates. A high-sugar meal with very little protein, such as a sweet roll and orange juice for breakfast, will have a different effect than one containing concentrated proteins like those from animal sources, legumes, or a complete protein combination such as oatmeal and soy milk.

Moreover, the effects of breakfast are even more pronounced on brain function than other meals, because we haven't eaten for several hours when we come to breakfast. Therefore, a mixed protein and complex carbohydrate breakfast is very important for those with AD/HD. For this reason, *leftovers from dinner*, which are often higher in protein, *make excellent breakfasts*.

During the postdigestive process, insulin is rapidly diverting glucose away from the brain. This effect is most pronounced when the meal contains little protein. We experience this as tiredness after a high-carbohydrate meal. The higher the sugar composition of the meal, the more likely we are to become tired. Two processes are at work here.

First, the brain compensates for lowered glucose levels by activating norepinephrine, which halts the flow of glucose away from the brain. Norepinephrine, a brain chemical that increases alertness and concentration, comes from protein foods and is readily available when the meal contains protein. If it does not, sufficient norepinephrine may not be available and we become less alert.

Second, insulin selects specific amino acids digested from protein for uptake in the liver and muscles and, in doing so, shifts the balance between brain chemicals. Another of these brain chemicals, *serotonin*, makes us sleepy and increases in concentration in the brain as norepinephrine is declining, which shifts brain activity from alert to sleepy.

Ultimately a vicious cycle is set up as the brain demands more glucose: we eat more sugar, then insulin kicks in, further lowering glucose levels. The AD/HD sufferer who chooses sugar may calm his brain down, an effect of serotonin, but he will also decrease his attention span and increase his mood swings—even depression. For some people, hyperactivity is a natural response to the lower glucose levels, as we have seen. Their bodies try to raise norepinephrine levels through movement, and the muscles have been well primed by insulin, which has moved extra glucose and amino acids into storage in these tissues.

In the meantime, the brain struggles to maintain communication between neurons, but the messages become unclear and confusing, making it impossible for a person experiencing this dynamic to concentrate. Another event now takes place in the brain as it builds up glucose deficits.

GLUCOSE EFFECTS ON NEUROTRANSMITTERS

A sugary meal causes a rise in glucose storage outside the brain and a shift in neurotransmitters, the chemical messengers that regulate the flow of information between neurons. In a tiny space between neurons, called the synapse, more than forty neurotransmitters are at work. The four most important in our discussion of AD/HD are *norepinephrine* and *dopamine*, also called *catecholamines*, which speed up the rate at which one neuron signals another; *acetylcholine*, which amplifies the signal being sent; and *serotonin*, which slows it down. By means of these four and the other neurotransmitters in the synapse, the brain controls the speed, intensity, and selectivity of messages being communicated.

Glucose metabolism in the brain dramatically affects the balance between the catecholamines and serotonin. High levels can slow down brain function as serotonin rises, but uneven distribution of energy from glucose also reduces brain activity as neurons struggle to process information.

Thus, when you already have a genetic error of metabolism—as it is now believed a significant number of AD/HD individuals do—consuming more sugar is a sure way to exaggerate the brain's malfunction. My *30-Day Plan* includes strategies to remove sugar from the diet and selectively use

ENLARGEMENT OF CONNECTION BETWEEN
AXON OF ONE NEURON AND DENDRITE OF ANOTHER

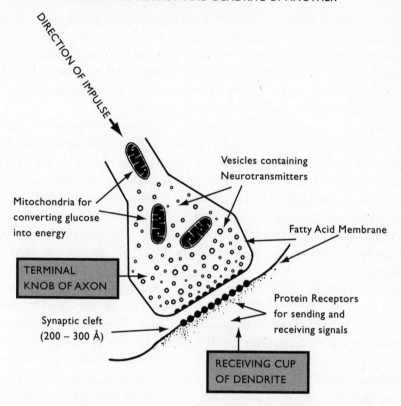

DIRECTION OF IMPULSE ➤

Vesicles containing
Neurotransmitters

Mitochondria for
converting glucose
into energy

Fatty Acid Membrane

TERMINAL
KNOB OF AXON

Protein Receptors
for sending and
receiving signals

Synaptic cleft
(200 – 300 Å)

RECEIVING CUP
OF DENDRITE

Energy from the mitochondria drives the neurotransmitter vesicles toward the sending proteins.
Neurotransmitters are released into the synaptic cleft. Mineral channels on the dendrite select
which neurotransmitters will be picked up by the protein receptors on the dendrite. Extra
neurotransmitters left in the synapse will be taken back into the terminal knob (reuptake).

complex carbohydrates to break the vicious cycle created by rapidly rising
glucose levels. We must achieve a good balance between complex carbohydrates, proteins, and fats to restore optimum brain function.

Carbohydrates provide fuel for our bodies, especially the brain, which
cannot break down either fats or proteins. In overcoming AD/HD, therefore, we must carefully plan the *type* of carbohydrates we eat and *when* we
eat them. Let's distinguish between the various types of carbohydrates.

TYPES OF CARBOHYDRATES

Simple sugars come into the diet from two sources, either those found naturally in fruit, fruit juices, dried fruit, fruit concentrates, and syrups, or those synthetically produced from corn, sugar beets, or sugarcane. Natural syrups include honey, maple, molasses, rice bran, and sorghum. All simple sugars, regardless of source, raise blood glucose levels quickly, and your body responds with a rapid production of insulin.

Foods that contain simple sugars are processed foods, such as candy, ice cream, jam, jellies, and condiments like ketchup and steak sauce. We rarely eat a teaspoon of sugar straight, although we add it liberally to beverages like coffee and iced tea. Over time this adds up. It is estimated that the average American eats 120 pounds of sugar each year. Most of the sugar comes from the processed foods and condiments that we consume, perhaps without realizing we are doing so. These sugary foods are wreaking havoc on our health but are especially deadly for AD/HD sufferers.

Natural sugars are considered more acceptable because they come from foods, rather than being synthesized, and are accompanied by other nutrients in the food that assist their assimilation. However, sugar-sensitive bodies do not tolerate these natural sugars any better than those from highly processed foods. Those with AD/HD are usually quite sugar-sensitive, which is why the *30-Day Plan* removes all forms of synthetic sugar and reduces use of natural sugars to a minimum. AD/HD individuals with yeast *(Candida)* overgrowth stemming from overuse of antibiotics will have to eliminate even natural sugars until they can reestablish normal intestinal flora.

As you observe the response you or your child has to natural sugars, you can decide if these foods must be eliminated from your diet as well. Many individuals with AD/HD have a marked inability to process sugars, and they experience severe drops in blood glucose levels two to three hours after eating that leave them shaky, dizzy, weak, and confused. This condition is known as *hypoglycemia* and requires extra vigilance in carbohydrate intake.

The best type of carbohydrates to eat are complex carbohydrates, which slowly release glucose into the system, slowing down the release of insulin and thereby preventing its action in diverting brain glucose. A complex carbohydrate is composed of starches—large molecules of several sugars combined—and fiber. Grains, beans, pasta, and vegetables all contain complex carbohydrates. Complex carbohydrates provide needed glucose without causing a rapid release of insulin and upsetting brain chemistry. Simple carbohydrates, in contrast, consist of sugars like glucose, sucrose, (table sugar), lactose (milk sugar), fructose, or corn syrup.

Whole grains contain the outer layer and inner germ of the grain as well as the starchy core. They also contain protein, essential fatty acids, vitamins, and minerals needed to digest and metabolize the grain. These are more desirable than refined carbohydrates because they come naturally with these essential nutrients.

Refining whole grains strips the outer layers, the bran, the germ, and most of the protein, fatty acids, vitamins, and minerals. To partly compensate for these losses, some of the B vitamins and one or two minerals are added back to "enriched" flours and cereal grains. Chromium is one of the trace minerals that is not added back, and it is a necessary element for your body to shuttle glucose into cells. Chromium makes insulin more efficient, thereby reducing the amount it takes to get glucose into your body cells. You are sure to get enough of this essential mineral if you follow the *30-Day Plan*.

We have seen that there are two sides to the carbohydrate picture. On the one hand, they provide necessary energy for your body, but on the other hand, they can disrupt brain function. We have also seen that the best choice for meeting these energy requirements is to choose complex carbohydrates from whole grains rather than anything made from refined flours or simple sugars. The next step is to choose the best time of day to eat carbohydrates in order to most benefit brain function.

WHEN CHILDREN SHOULD EAT CARBOHYDRATES

Several investigations have been made into the effects of meal composition on school performance. According to Bonnie Spring, Ph.D., a researcher in the department of psychology at Texas Tech University, in Lubbock, Texas, the most significant effects were seen after breakfast. Children who ate a high-carbohydrate breakfast scored more poorly on tests of attention than children who had no breakfast at all! Those who had eaten a high-protein breakfast did much better than those who either ate no breakfast or ate one rich in carbohydrates.

Moreover, the children who ate a high-carbohydrate breakfast were affected quickly, within thirty minutes after they ate. The effect lasted for four hours. In other words, if your child eats a high-carbohydrate breakfast without a balance of protein, his mind may be under siege all morning. If he then eats a high-carbohydrate or sugary lunch, the effect can last the entire school day. In the clinical trials, the effects seen after a high-carbohydrate lunch were not as dramatic as those seen after a high carbohydrate breakfast. Yet carbohydrates, which raise serotonin levels, can have a dramatic impact on brain function in children. What about adults with AD/HD?

HOW CARBOHYDRATES AFFECT ADULTS

Similar tests run on adults failed to find such a clear-cut response to carbohydrates, although many adults have learned to mix and match proteins and carbohydrates for clearer thinking and smoother energy response. In an adult study reviewed by Bonnie Spring, Ph.D., and published in *Nutrition and the Brain*, carbohydrate-rich meals produced significantly greater sleepiness 2 hours after being consumed than did protein-rich meals. Many adults reported "calming effects" from eating carbohydrates, presumably because serotonin levels were raised. One research team noted that women will change carbohydrate and protein choices depending on their menstrual cycle. Carbohydrates that raise serotonin levels are preferred just prior to menstruation.

Nevertheless, the reported glucose impairment in the frontal lobes of AD/HD adults can seriously affect mental performance, since the frontal lobe handles mental representations involved in cognition, ideas, and abstractions. If sugar metabolism is disturbed in those with AD/HD, how is it affected by artificial sweeteners? Are they a healthy, helpful option?

ASPARTAME—SWEET PROMISES

I was enthusiastic at first when the sweetener aspartame, registered under the trade names NutraSweet and Equal, was introduced in the early 1980s. It was expected there would be few if any side effects caused by aspartame, since it is made from the amino acids *phenylalanine* and *aspartic acid*, which your body needs. Phenylalanine is an essential amino acid, one that must be supplied daily because your body can't manufacture it. It is the precursor of two of the major neurotransmitters discussed above, namely norepinephrine and dopamine. The amino acid aspartic acid is also an important excitatory neurotransmitter, although the body can manufacture it.

A tasteless sweetener with no calories, which could be safely used by those who react to sugar, seemed too good to be true . . . and it was. Shortly after its introduction into foods, the Centers for Disease Control published the results of a 1983 study they conducted on consumer-based complaints associated with food products containing aspartame. Complaints involved upsets to the central nervous and digestive systems and gynecological problems.

Reported central nervous system symptoms included mood changes, insomnia, and seizures. Gastrointestinal complaints included abdominal pain, nausea, and diarrhea. Irregular menses was the single gynecological complaint reported.

To illustrate how severe these symptoms can be, here is a case reported in the scientific literature. It involved a teenage girl who discovered her sensitivity to NutraSweet. She was extremely popular, athletic, and had excellent grades, but like many teenage girls she became obsessed with her weight. So she decided to switch to diet beverages sweetened with NutraSweet. At first she consumed one or two per day, but she quickly increased her intake to several each day because she enjoyed the "high" they gave her.

After a few weeks of drinking several diet beverages a day, her behavior began to change dramatically. She was less agile, became moody, and had difficulty sustaining her grade point average. Her friends noticed that she became irritable, short tempered, and argumentative.

During the summer break, she went away to cheerleader camp for a week. No diet drinks were available. After an initial two days of feeling lethargic and having headaches, she began to feel better. By the end of the week she felt better than she had in months, and her friends noticed a complete reversal of her symptoms. Upon her return home, she sampled a diet beverage and immediately became depressed and lethargic. Suspecting a reaction to the NutraSweet, she withdrew diet beverages for a few days and then tried them again, with the same results. Now she was certain of her sensitivity to aspartame, and she has avoided it ever since. How, then, does NutraSweet affect the brain?

William Pardridge, M.D., of the UCLA Department of Medicine, explained its effects in a paper entitled "Potential Effects of the Dipeptide Sweetener Aspartame on the Brain," published in *Nutrition and the Brain*, volume 7. As we have seen, aspartame consists of the amino acids aspartic acid and phenylalanine. Because of the protective blood brain barrier, the entry of aspartic acid is slowed down and its effects appear to be minimal.

However, phenylalanine readily crosses the blood brain barrier and is converted within the neurons into the excitatory neurotransmitters norepinephrine and dopamine. If the blood is delivering more phenylalanine than other amino acids to the brain, the natural balance of neurotransmitters is upset. The neurotransmitters that are crowded out are the calming and stabilizing ones, serotonin and dopamine. As a result, symptoms that occur may include insomnia, short attention span, hyperactivity, behavioral changes, hormone changes, decreased agility, and seizures in those with a family history of this condition. No wonder the teenage girl described in the medical literature had these symptoms. She consumed as many as eight aspartame-laden drinks per day!

According to Dr. Pardridge, levels of phenylalanine high enough to push the upper limits of safety can occur if your child drinks a quart (four standard cans) or more per day of beverages containing NutraSweet. If your child is eating snacks containing NutraSweet or Equal, these may contribute even more of these potentially harmful ingredients to his diet.

In addition to the neurotransmitters, NutraSweet contains methanol, which must be metabolized by the liver in the same manner as ethanol, the alcohol found in wine, beer, and spirits. For adults consuming diet mixers with alcoholic drinks, the methanol in the mixer adds additional work for the liver. Methanol, sometimes called wood alcohol, is produced in small amounts by bacteria in the digestive system. Normally the amount produced is not harmful, but if enough additional methanol is ingested, the potential for toxicity, especially in children, is considerably increased.

Incredibly, in twenty years of testing, the developers of NutraSweet never checked to see what effects this chemical might have on the brain. Yet it was approved for use by the FDA before this was known, and they have approved several other artificial sweeteners that can detrimentally affect brain function as well.

ACESULFAME K: USE APPROVAL EXPANDED

Acesulfame K (acesulfame potassium), sold under the name Sunett, is an artificial sweetener two hundred times sweeter than sucrose or table sugar. Sunett is used in foods, beverages, tabletop sweeteners, pharmaceuticals, dietary supplements, including protein powders and nutrition bars, and cosmetics requiring a sweet taste. Sunett is extremely stable, making it suitable also for baked or frozen products. It isn't as fluffy as sugar and recipes using it must be revised, but otherwise it seems like a chemist's dream come true. Even though Sunett is sweeter than sugar, it contains no calories!

Like aspartame, saccharin, cyclamates, and other artificial sweeteners, Sunett is not metabolized as sugar. In fact, it's not metabolized at all, but passes unchanged from the body. While the tongue perceives it as intensely sweet, the digestive system doesn't recognize it and therefore cannot break it down.

Sunett was approved for dietary use in the late 1980s, just a few years after aspartame. However, most of us were not aware of its existence—why? If Sunett is used as the exclusive sweetening agent, it leaves an unpleasant bitter aftertaste on the tongue but it could still be used to substantially reduce the amount of sugar needed in sweetened foods, which would cut calories and make it a winner in the diet food category. However, there are questions about whether Sunett is safe, when consumed even in moderate amounts, and this limits its broad acceptance by the food industry.

The significant danger for those with AD/HD, however, is that Sunett stimulates insulin release even though it isn't metabolized by the body. The sweetness perceived in the mouth sends a powerful message to the pancreas to release insulin because a sugar meal is on the way! We can try to fool the body, but if insulin is released, the accompanying dampening effects on neurotransmitters occur.

SUCRALOSE: ANOTHER PROMISE OF SWEETNESS THAT DOESN'T DELIVER

The FDA approved another new sweetener, called sucralose, in May 1998. Splenda, the Canadian name, has been in use in Canada since 1991. This sweetener can be added to baked goods and foods that are to be heated to high temperatures. Thus, it has the potential of inclusion in even more foods than NutraSweet, which breaks down when it is heated. Sucralose has been approved for addition into all baked goods, baking mixes, nonalcoholic beverages, chewing gum, coffee and tea products, confections and frostings, fat and oils, frozen dairy desserts and mixes, fruit and water ices, gelatins, puddings and fillings, jams and jellies, milk products, processed fruits and fruit juices, sugar substitutes, sweet sauces, toppings, syrups, and as a tabletop sweetener.

Sucralose was originally produced in England in 1976 by two chemists who found that ordinary table sugar could be combined with chlorine gas to produce a complex chemical that the tongue detected as sweet with an intensity six hundred times that of sugar. It turns out that beyond its sweet promise, sucralose is so artificial, the body cannot recognize it and passes it up for absorption *as a nutrient*. However, it still goes to the liver, which must figure out what to do with it.

Since it can't be broken down, the liver treats sucralose as a *xenobiotic* or foreign chemical, one that must be detoxified by protective enzymes in the liver. The ultimate toxicity of sucralose rests on how difficult it is for these enzymes to get rid of it and what kind of by-products will be produced as a result. Experience has taught us that the potential toxicity of a chemical depends on whatever else the liver has had to process. *The more toxic food chemicals, inhalants, and drugs (prescription or OTC) the liver is confronted with, the greater the potential for toxic effects of artificial ingredients like sucralose.*

It's tempting to think you can eat all the sweet-tasting foods you want and not have any calories to count. But the reason it sounds too good to be true is that—to date—it is. This new sweetener may have the potential for doing even more harm than aspartame or acesulfame K.

The good news is that sucralose is less likely to promote cavities than sugar, because the bacteria in the mouth that cause dental caries cannot utilize it either. Sucralose also does not have the unpleasant aftertaste of acesulfame K. Although sucralose offers no substantial advantage over xylitol and sorbitol—the sweeteners commonly found in toothpastes—in cavity prevention, whereas the latter are metabolized because they are normally found in the body, sucralose is not. Therefore, sucralose may be an excellent addition to mouthwash, toothpaste, and other oral hygiene products that should taste good but never be swallowed.

ARTIFICIAL INDIGESTIBLE INGREDIENTS: PRESUMED INNOCENT?

Alpha-amylase inhibitors or starch blockers were popular in the mid-1980s because they blocked the digestion of carbohydrates, promising that you could eat as much pasta as you wanted without any calories. Americans rushed to try the newest weight-control gimmick, but so many people complained about stomachaches and other gastrointestinal upsets that the fad died before long.

Chitin from shellfish is another material that is not digested, but traps and removes dietary fats on its way through our digestive systems. This material toughens the shells of crustaceans like crabs, shrimp, and lobsters. The processed material, known by trade names such as Chitosan, traps fats before they can pass through the intestinal wall, thus preventing their absorption in the digestive system. Unfortunately, chitin can cause irritation to the digestive system and indiscriminately remove good as well as bad fats; it is therefore not used much at all.

OLESTRA—MORE TROUBLE

And now we have olestra, marketed under the name Olean and manufactured by Procter & Gamble. Olestra is a conglomerate of many sugar molecules tightly bound to fatty acids. This sugar/fat polymer is so big it

cannot pass intact through the intestinal wall, and so complex, that digestive enzymes cannot split the molecule into smaller, more absorbable
units. Your tongue will pick up the creaminess of fat and this causes a
pleasant taste sensation, but like acesulfame K, sucralose, and chitin,
olestra goes right through you . . . and drags along some important nutrients in the process that should be left for your body to absorb.

Olestra traps fat-soluble vitamins like vitamin A, vitamin D, vitamin E,
and the antioxidant carotenes that are waiting for passage into circulation
during the digestive process. The FDA was worried about the problem
this could cause, especially for children, but not worried enough to withhold approval of the material for use in snack foods. The FDA approval
was conditional upon Procter & Gamble advising its customers to fortify
all foods containing olestra with vitamins A, D, and E. However, no label
warning is required to advise consumers of the antivitamin activity of
olestra. Besides robbing the body of nutrients, olestra also interferes with
metabolism of essential fatty acids and fat-soluble antioxidants such as
beta-carotene, lycopene, lutein, and zeaxanthin, and you'll find out why
these are important in later chapters. Incredibly, the reported response of
the FDA, when confronted with this reality, was that fatty acids and
carotenoids haven't been established as vitamins and therefore are of less
concern.

Olestra was test-marketed in several U.S. cities. Snack items containing olestra were made freely available to citizens in a city in Iowa, and
the initial response was very favorable. In a few hours, however, many
local citizens who had sampled several of the snacks suddenly suffered
distressing bouts of diarrhea. One could only hope similar episodes occur
frequently enough to limit use of this product! Obviously, I do not recommend this product to anyone, let alone those with AD/HD. I do not
recommend buying products with any of these artificial ingredients in
them, because they disturb glucose and fatty acid metabolism, both of
which are vital to brain function.

EFFECTS OF PROTEINS ON THE BRAIN

Proteins contain twenty or more amino acids, of which eight are considered essential, or must be eaten daily, and two as semiessential for adults
but essential for children. Amino acids are the basic units of growth,
building muscles, organs, and other tissues of our bodies. They are also
essential for brain function.

When we eat proteins, more norepinephrine and dopamine are available than serotonin. That's because tyrosine and phenylalanine, which

yield dopamine and norepinephrine, are more plentiful in proteins than tryptophan, one of the eight essential amino acids, which yields serotonin. These three amino acids compete for delivery to the brain, and tryptophan, being less concentrated, loses out. Even when high-tryptophan-containing foods such as dairy products or turkey are eaten, tyrosine and phenylalanine still have the advantage.

Recall for a moment what I said earlier, that tryptophan will be picked up and concentrated best when carbohydrate foods are eaten along with proteins. This is the reason for timing meal content as I do in my *30-Day Plan. We can think of proteins as fuel for thought and carbohydrates as good for promoting drowsiness.*

Amino acids also function in many ways that are just as important to brain function as neurotransmitters. They make up the enzymes that regulate neurotransmitters. Without these enzymes, neurons could not receive, process, interpret, and output vital information. Any amino acid or small protein that has an effect on the transmission of information between neurons is called a neurotransmitter. What are some of these, and how does what we eat affect their levels in the brain?

OTHER NEUROTRANSMITTERS: EFFECTS

Overcoming AD/HD, especially in children, necessitates consumption of a high percentage (30 percent of daily calories) of good, high-quality proteins such as fish, poultry, lamb, pork, and beef, as well as organically grown vegetables, legumes such as soybeans and peas, and whole grains.

Allergies and food sensitivities must be considered when we discuss proteins because they can also play a major role in symptoms of AD/HD. These symptoms also interfere with good digestion and impede the effective delivery of amino acids into the system. According to Jon Pangborn, Ph.D., who has reviewed thousands of laboratory tests on individuals with AD/HD, poor protein digestion is a common factor in those suffering from food allergies. When proteins are improperly digested, large peptide units pass into the system and trigger an immune response. Not only that, if proteins are not properly digested, they cannot yield the amino acids needed for neurotransmitters. They may even yield toxic byproducts that can slow down mental processing and further compromise the immune system. Therefore, it is necessary to address this potential problem by using digestive enzymes that ensure efficient delivery of the needed amino acids to the brain. My *30-Day Plan* provides these digestive enzymes.

Acetylcholine (AC) is the neurotransmitter associated with memory and efficient cognition. Choline, the main constituent of acetylcholine, is also a component of *phosphatidyl choline* or PC. PC is one of four phosphatides that act like Velcro on the surface of neurons and other cells in your body. They grab messages that are being transferred between neurons and are the attachments for the essential fatty acids.

Both dietary and supplemental choline must be available to become well absorbed and utilized in the manufacture of both acetylcholine and PC if our thought processes are to flow quickly and smoothly. Disruption of acetylcholine activity has not been demonstrated in AD/HD, although it has been in memory disorders. Of importance in AD/HD is the role choline plays as PC and its stress-rebound ability. PC is the base attachment of arachidonic acid, the second most important fatty acid in the brain.

Acetylcholine is classified as a "cholinergic" neurotransmitter—one that is opposite in action from the catecholamines. AC amplifies messages being sent across the synapse, while the catecholamines speed the rate of transmission. We experience a shift between these neurotransmitters as quick thinking and responsiveness (catecholamines) and contemplation (acetylcholine). We need a balance of both. During stressful periods, we selectively drive our neurons with catecholamines. Catecholamine activity keeps us sharp, but we usually experience less depth to our thoughts. Our bodies need to recoup with periods of selecting acetylcholine to restore mental balance.

Can we increase the yield of acetylcholine by dietary change? The answer is yes, and the use of soy foods in my *30-Day Plan* increases the amount of choline available to the brain. The foods that contain large amounts of choline are liver, oatmeal, soy foods, cauliflower, kale, and cabbage. The granular lecithin that I add to my "Power Shake" also provides choline.

It is important to note that acetylcholine, phosphatidyl choline, and the other important phosphatide, phosphatidyl serine, are all present in significant levels in human breast milk. Nature has supplied the perfect balance of phosphatides and fatty acids needed for development of the baby's brain. These building blocks for a healthy brain are very important to the developing child. This is just another reason why mothers should breast-feed their children if possible.

FATS, FATTY ACIDS, AND AD/HD

We have been repeatedly warned about the dangers of a high-fat diet; it is believed to contribute to the major chronic diseases of our day, and rightly so. However, the message has gotten confused. Americans have also confused cholesterol with fat, often considering them as one and the same. However, as medical experts have learned more about the role of cholesterol in heart disease, they have modified their stand. Now we know that the kind of cholesterol present, low-density lipoproteins (LDL) or high-density lipoproteins (HDL), is as important as total cholesterol. HDL is considered the good kind, while LDL is considered the bad one and an indicator of future cardiovascular disease. Furthermore, many of the processed fats we once thought were good for us are no longer considered so. The result is a vigorous debate over the most widely consumed spreads—butter and margarine. The medical community needs to clarify this message about fats. Which ones *are* good for you?

According to results obtained from the ongoing Boston Nurses Health Study, there is good reason to worry about the artificial fats found in margarine, fast foods, French fries, doughnuts, crackers, and commercial baked goods. In assessing the effects on eighty thousand nurses of the "bad" fats found in these foods, a crucial factor in the development of heart disease has been identified. Researchers now think the risk from consuming these fats is greater than that from smoking and high blood pressure. The result? Please pass the butter!

As for the current love affair we Americans have for *fat-free*, the creamy texture and taste we have come to love is now replaced in many processed foods by sugars of various forms. Actually when we eat them we wind up sabotaging our efforts to reduce fat accumulation in our bodies. When introduced to our systems in excess, these sugars are converted and stored—you guessed it—as fat! In addition, some of the weight gain that is occurring in this country's population *since our awareness of the dangers of fats* has come from people thinking of fat-free items as ones they can eat much more of than their fat-filled equivalent. This is just not true. We have made some beneficial changes to our diets over the last three years, but there still is a long way to go.

AD/HD STRATEGIES

Now it's time to discuss the specific *30-Day Program* that will help curtail AD/HD symptoms. This will involve the introduction of a certain number of servings of each food group daily as recommended by age and gender. I outline specific guidelines in the following pages that will make it simple for you to make quick and easy dietary changes.

Many find that the biggest hurdle they face in making any health-conscious dietary adjustments is substituting new foods into family menu plans. To overcome this, you should try to focus on the positive behavioral changes that are your goal. In addition, you can share with your family the excitement that comes from embarking on new taste adventures. Do remember, however, that the younger your children are, the easier your adjustment will be. Try to incorporate a wide variety of healthy foods into your children's diet as early as you can—preferably when they are still in the high chair. We all tend to choose a few favorite foods, with the result that we miss many important nutrients and may even develop an addiction or allergy to these foods due to repeated exposure. Eating as varied a diet as possible provides us with the full range of nutrients we need. Scientists have noted that animals instinctively select as wide a range of foods as possible, and we should do the same.

Today you can purchase peaches, grapes, tomatoes, and apples all year round in most markets. Improved transportation and storage methods make most foods available year round, making it easy to cater to our selective tastes. Grapes and tomatoes are shipped in from Chile and other countries close to the Equator and we can have them spring, summer, winter, or fall, if we like.

However, any of you who grew up on or around farms remember how wonderful it was to eat fruits and vegetables in season. When the first peaches and apricots ripened, we climbed up into the trees and gorged ourselves. I can still remember the sensation of juice running down my arms. By the end of the season, we were sick of peaches, and the mere thought of peach fuzz made us itch! Then the season changed, and we eagerly went after some other seasonal fruit like grapes, pomegranates, persimmons, or apples.

Until rather recently, seasonal changes necessitated dietary changes when our fruits and vegetables came only from local farms, and the possibility of building up intolerance to specific foods was greatly reduced. Today we don't have the seasonal limitations on our diets that we once did, and we can easily diversify our diet by choosing new and exotic foods that are unfamiliar to those of us who were raised on regional American cuisine. Most of us have gone into restaurants that serve dishes native to other countries and enjoyed what we ate. Now we can serve many of these dishes at home. In our attempt to eat a healthy variety of foods we have a much larger number of meats, fruits, vegetables, and grains to choose from, so at the very least we can add some fun new foods to our diet.

WHY EATING ORGANIC FOODS IS BETTER

Most people who choose to buy organic foods instead of commercial grade do so because they want to decrease the amount of pesticides, herbicides, and other chemicals they eat. This is a good reason to eat organically. However, another reason to spend the time and money it takes to find good organic food is that it often tastes better. Organic fruits and vegetables are usually grown locally and arrive to the market with less time and handling between the field and the shelf than commercially grown produce. Freshness alone will improve the flavor and nutritional content.

I have noted in charts how many servings of each food are recommended for people of different ages. By making daily food choices with these guidelines in mind, you will help alleviate AD/HD symptoms that are diet related, and you will enjoy some new taste treats.

VEGETABLES

Mother Nature has provided foods with specific nutrients that support seasonal resistance to disease. We can best take advantage of nature's plan by eating foods in season and from areas as close to home as possible. Traditional wisdom has held this to be true, and now scientific research is providing reasons why this practice is important. Fruits and vegetables contain phytochemicals—nutrients beyond vitamins and minerals—that have many health-promoting and disease-preventing benefits.

We can put science into practice by eating foods in season, when the phytochemical content is highest and can offer the best protection. Foods available in winter, for example, are rich in carotenoids and complex carbohydrates. These include winter squash, sweet potatoes, yams, carrots, Swiss chard, spinach, and other dark greens. They provide antioxidant protection against infections that more commonly occur in winter. Complex carbohydrates provide energy as heat, which we need just to keep warm at this time of year.

Tomatoes, on the other hand, are an example of the perfect summer vegetable. They are rich in lycopene, a carotenoid that protects the skin from ultraviolet light in the hotter months. The more ripening that occurs on the vine, the more lycopene tomatoes contain. We can enjoy tomatoes all year round, but fresh tomatoes are best eaten in the summer when they are naturally in season. Dried, canned, or bottled varieties can be eaten other times of the year. The dried and canned varieties have been harvested and processed at the peak of their ripeness and have concentrated levels of lycopene. Fresh tomatoes available out of season are likely to have been gassed to color them up, but the intense red color that signals high lycopene content is usually absent. However, while tomatoes are a great addition to most diets, avoid eating them several times a week because you may become sensitized to them, and certainly don't eat them if you have an allergy to them.

Brassica (cruciferous) vegetables include broccoli, cauliflower, bok choy, Brussels sprouts, cabbage, kale, and mustard. These vegetables contain sulfur phytochemicals and vitamin C that boost the body's detoxifying processes. We can eat them all year round in cooler climate areas where they grow. But, when in doubt, always try to eat what is in season, grown locally and organic if possible, for your best vegetable value.

Cooking Tips

Vegetables are the most exciting foods we can eat. They come in every color of the rainbow and add endless variety to meals. Plan rainbow meals; combine foods for their color and you will provide the best array of nutrients for your body. Children generally like vegetables because they are colorful and easy to eat. Preparation is the key to enjoying them.

Cook your vegetables soon after you bring them home. The nutrient content is highest then, and you will cut down on waste. The cooked vegetables will keep several days in your refrigerator. Children will snack on stored vegetables if they are readily available, and it is easy to toss cooked veggies into dishes just before serving. Busy people do not need the added pressure to use up stored veggies before they go bad.

If you are going to stir-fry your veggies, use cooking spray to cut down on the oil you are using. Also, if you are using the firmer vegetables, steam or blanch them ahead of time so you can add them last. This will make your finished stir-fry more attractive and appealing.

Soft, leafy vegetables taste good raw or very lightly sautéed or steamed. Tomatoes, peppers, celery, and some root vegetables are delicious when raw. Firm vegetables are more palatable if they are lightly cooked, preferably steamed, just until they are tender and still brightly colored. Carotenoid phytochemicals are easier to obtain when vegetables that contain them are lightly steamed. Winter squash, yams, sweet potatoes, and pumpkin should be cooked, usually baked, until soft.

Daily Servings Guide

Vegetables provide most of the vitamins, minerals, and phytochemicals we get in our diet. They are extremely important for brain and nervous system function.

AGE	NUMBER OF VEGETABLE SERVINGS ½ cup each, (size of a tennis ball or a single ice-cream scoop)
1–3 years	3
4–6 years	4
7–10 years	5
11–14 years	6
Girls 15 through adult	6
Pregnant 2nd & 3rd trimesters	6

AGE	NUMBER OF VEGETABLE SERVINGS ½ cup each, (size of a tennis ball or a single ice-cream scoop)
Lactating	8
Teenage boys	7
Men 19 through adult	8

Does this sound like a lot? Follow my easy menu plans and you will find it is easy to meet these requirements. Six or eight servings of vegetables can easily be reached with a large helping of steamed vegetables and a good-sized green salad.

OILS AND FATS

Oils and fats are classified as *lipids,* and both have developed a bad reputation. Recently, the American Heart Association has taken a different position on these fats. While scientists and the Heart Association still caution about overeating fats, they are emphasizing the need to avoid the bad fats. The reasons for this are simple. When solid fats—the bad ones—are added to the diet, cholesterol in the blood increases. On the other hand, when liquid unsaturated and polyunsaturated oils replace solid fats, cholesterol decreases. However, in spite of this reality, many of us have understood the message as "avoid *all* fats," the good and the bad. We have substituted fat-free replacements for favorite snack foods.

Experts testified at a February 1998 convention on diet and heart disease in San Francisco that Americans have enthusiastically embraced fat-free foods, but they are adding extra servings of carbohydrates as a result. The experts cautioned against this practice because, ultimately, the extra carbohydrates will be stored as fat, and that is just as bad for your heart as eating fats in the first place.

You must be smart about fat, especially where children are concerned. Do not feed them a low-fat diet, because they need the good fats for brain development. Which fats should you choose and which should you avoid when shopping for and preparing meals?

All lipids are classified as hydrocarbons because they contain only carbon and hydrogen. Carbon makes up the lipid backbone, with hydrogen atoms filling some or all of the empty spaces along the backbone. If only some spaces are filled, the fat is unsaturated. If all the spaces are filled, it is saturated, or some sites may remain unoccupied. Consequently the lipid is not saturated.

The hydrogen saturation of the carbon imparts a fixed, rigid structure that makes saturated fats solid at room temperature. Beef fat is an example of a saturated fat—the kind you should try to limit in your diet. Unsaturated and polyunsaturated fats have spaces between the carbon atoms where there are no hydrogen atoms, lending flexibility to the lipid, and they remain liquid even when refrigerated. Safflower, sunflower, flaxseed, and other vegetable oils are examples of unsaturated fats that are healthier for you than saturated fats.

Monounsaturated fats have carbon backbones with a single open space. They are the best kind of dietary fat to buy because they are more stable, less likely to turn rancid, and actually help your body to decrease cholesterol. Olive and canola oils are mono-unsaturated and are your best choices for salad dressings, cooking, and baking.

The oils in fish are unsaturated because fish live in cold temperatures that would turn their body oils solid if they were saturated. Fish oils have many health-promoting benefits and are the best dietary sources of the unsaturated fats your body needs for brain and body cells. When you eat fish, especially those from deep cold water, you get custom-designed oils that are immediately available to your own brain cells and your cardiovascular and other body systems. The best fish oils come from salmon, herring, cod, and menhaden. These oils contain *zoochemicals*, the animal equivalent of fruit and vegetable phytochemicals. Fish oils are available as dietary supplements, with concentrated amounts of zoochemicals, and are one of the keys to success with my *30-Day Plan*.

Hydrogenated fats are made from unsaturated oils by forcing hydrogen atoms into some open spaces between carbons. Consequently, they are solid at room temperature. Heat and pressure are required to hydrogenate oils, and this produces harmful fats called *trans* fats. Scientists have implicated trans fats with some types of cancer. The February 1998 issue of *The Harvard Health Letter* discussed the butter/margarine controversy: "The ongoing Nurses Health Study . . . provide(s) further evidence that so-called *trans fats*—found in margarine, commercially baked goods (crackers, cookies, cakes), and many deep-fried foods—promote heart disease." Shortening, margarine, hydrogenated cottonseed oil, and palm kernel oils are all hydrogenated fats that should be avoided. These fats are especially bad for those with AD/HD because they block the enzymes in the body that reconfigure dietary unsaturated fats into the longer-chain polyunsaturated fats needed for brain function. Researchers have found that those with AD/HD had lower levels of these important brain fats than those without the disorders.

BEST OILS TO CHOOSE

Here is the nutritional profile for monounsaturated oils:

SUPER CANOLA OIL*

Nutrition Facts
Serving Size 1 Tbs. (14 g.)
Amount Per Serving
Calories 120 Calories from Fat

	% of Daily Value†
Total Fat 14 g.	22%
Saturated Fat (the bad kind), 1 gram	
Polyunsaturated Fat (better kind), 2 grams	
Monounsaturated Fat (best kind), 11 grams	
Cholesterol, 0 mg	0%
Sodium, 0 mg	0%
Total Carbohydrates, 0 mg	0%
Total Protein, 0 mg	0%

*Not a significant source of dietary fiber, sugars, vitamin A, vitamin C, calcium, and iron.
†Percent Daily Values are based on a 2,000 calorie diet.

Both canola and extravirgin olive oils contain a high level of mono-unsaturated fat, which makes them more stable and not as likely to turn rancid. Refrigerate these oils, even though olive oil will harden slightly, making it somewhat inconvenient to use without first letting it warm to room temperature. You can work around this problem by storing a small amount in a cruet topped with vitamin E oil, which will protect it from going bad. Keep it in a cool, dark cupboard ready for use.

BEST SPREAD TO USE

Butter is a better choice than margarine or shortening. It is a saturated fat, but contains no harmful trans fats. Butter needs to be used sparingly because it is saturated, but you can improve its nutrition and spreadability by making "Sunshine Butter." This is a blend of unsalted butter, canola oil, and a bit of vitamin E oil for stability. I'll tell you how to make this in the recipe section.

NUT AND SEED BUTTERS AND OILS

More of these "exotic" oils are becoming available in markets. They add variety to salad dressings and different flavors for cooking. These oils consist mostly of unsaturated and monounsaturated oils with few saturated fats.

Butters made from ground seeds and nuts are also becoming increasingly available. Children are likely to have allergic reactions to peanuts and peanut butter, especially if consumed often. You can substitute almond, sesame, or cashew butter for peanut butter to try and avoid this reaction. These spreads are delicious on toast or crackers.

Nut butters, like nut oils, contain mostly unsaturated fats. Think of them as substitutes for butter or other high-fat spreads as you add them into menu plans. They also contain proteins and carbohydrates. The protein content of nut butters is around 19 percent of the total calories in the spread, while carbohydrates account for 13 percent. Therefore, they offer more balanced nutrition than butter for AD/HD children. Sesame butter and sesame tahini are good sources of calcium as well. All nut butters and their oils should be stored in the refrigerator. If your market doesn't stock these items yet, a nearby health food store will. I have also included a list of mail-order houses in appendix 2 for your ordering convenience.

Restrict butter, cream, cream cheese, and bacon in your child's diet because they are high in saturated fats. I suggest you do not use margarine at all because it contains saturated and trans fats. Reduced-calorie or low-fat spreads usually substitute various forms of sugar and aren't a better choice for that reason. Two-thirds of your daily servings of fats should be oils (canola, olive, safflower, soy) and as much as one-third can be saturated fats.

DAILY SERVINGS GUIDE

AGE	NUMBER OF OIL AND FAT SERVINGS
1–3 years	3
4–6 years	5
7–10 years	5
11–14 years	
girls	5
boys	6

AGE	NUMBER OF OIL AND FAT SERVINGS
girls 15 through adult	5
pregnant 2nd & 3rd trimesters	6
lactating	7
teenage boys	6
men 19 through adult	7

Each serving equals:
one teaspoon of oil, butter, or mayonnaise, or
two teaspoons of ranch, bleu cheese, or thousand island dressing, or
one tablespoon of nut butter, salad dressing, or cream cheese, or
one slice of bacon, or
two tablespoons of cream or sour cream, or
one-eighth of an avocado, or ten small or five large olives

BEVERAGES

I suggest you begin substituting soy milk for cow's milk in recipes and offer it to your children as another beverage option. Let them become used to it, find out their favorite flavors, and then you can gradually reduce the amount of cow's milk they drink. Soy milk is becoming available in many stores, plain or flavored. Unflavored soy milk is the best choice for cooking. The flavored varieties are tastier and will no doubt be a better beverage choice for your family. It is best to buy organic soy beverages whenever possible, to avoid pesticides and chemicals commonly used on soy crops.

Nutritionally, soy milk is close to whole milk; in addition it contains fiber, which milk does not. The principal benefit for AD/HD individuals in substituting soy milk for cow's milk, however, is reduction of their allergic response. For years, pediatricians have been prescribing soy formula for infants with milk intolerance. My first experience with soy beverages was my younger brother's soy formula which, when I tried it, sent terrible signals to my childish taste buds. Consequently, I was slow to try the new soy beverages as an adult. I was curious, however, why they were so popular with children, and I was pleasantly surprised to find out how tasty they really can be.

Occasionally, a child will have allergies to both cow's milk and soy milk. Fortunately, this is not often the case. If your child is allergic to both of these, substitute rice or nut beverages and be sure to include the calcium supplement I am recommending. You will also have to check labels on brands recommended in the Pantry Management section of my book to avoid soy.

Substituting soy milk for cow's milk in your child's diet does mean a change in the nutrients he or she is receiving. One cup of soy milk provides 4 percent of your child's daily requirement for calcium, much lower than he or she would get in the same serving of cow's milk. However, I am recommending you supplement this important brain mineral anyway, as part of my *30-Day Plan*. The up side is that soy milk does contain 20 percent of your child's daily requirement for vitamin A and one-third of his iron requirement. In addition, soy products contain a remarkable phytochemical that was shown to boost immune system activity in two recent studies published in *Nutrition and Cancer*. One way it does this is by increasing the number and bacteria/viral killing activity of macrophages and lymphocytes, two kinds of scavenging white blood cells. The other is by increasing a chemical released by the immune system, called interleukin, which orchestrates immune response. Another added benefit that soy provides is a boost to the weight of the thymus gland, which is located under the breastbone. This gland produces immune system cells.

Adults can benefit from adding soy products to their dietary program because they contain phytochemicals called *isoflavones*. These substances are believed by scientists to reduce the incidence of breast and prostate cancers. The earlier one starts eating soy products, the better—according to a recent study published in *Carcinogenesis*. Isoflavones compete with estrogen by locking up estrogen receptors in breast tissue before estrogen can attach itself and cause possible harm. Asian women who eat soy foods for a lifetime are virtually free of breast cancer as well as the discomfort that can come from the body's estrogen reduction that occurs during menopause, such as hot flashes.

Rice milk is another beverage that can be added to your child's diet, for a break from milk. Although rice milk does not supply the same nutrition as milk, it is light and sweet and children find its taste very appealing. Rice milk is ideal for my Power Shake recipe, particularly as a substitute for juice, and it goes along nicely in the lunch box. Rice milk is lower in protein and fat than regular milk, higher in carbohydrates, and contains 2 percent of the daily requirement for calcium. Rice milk made from organic brown rice is the best choice because it contains vitamin E and phytochemicals called *tocotrienols*. Researchers have shown several unique cardiovascular benefits of tocotrienols, including reduction of blood lipid and cholesterol levels and reduction of a protein called apolipoprotein B that contributes to heart disease.

Nut milks are another alternative to cow's milk. Nut milks are made by mixing ground nuts with boiling water in a blender or food processor. They are best made ahead so the nutty flavor permeates the liquid. They store nicely for several days in the refrigerator. Use three parts noncarbonated or spring water to each part ground nuts. If you use almonds, you may want to remove the skins first. Do this by dropping them into a pan of boiling water, turning off the heat, and letting the nuts sit in the water until the skins puff. Pour off the hot water, let the nuts cool until you can easily handle them, then pop the whole nuts from the loose skins by squeezing on the wider end.

Fruit juices are favorite beverages for kids. However, they contain natural sugars without the fiber of whole fruit to slow the body's metabolism of the fruit sugars. For this reason they can be a significant source of irritation to AD/HD children. I do not recommend orange, apple, or grape juice. This is primarily because they appear overfrequently in children's foods, and because they are high in sugars. Try pineapple, papaya, guava, apricot, peach, and pear juices instead.

Vegetable juices are an even better choice. They contain proteins and carbohydrates plus a little fiber to assist carbohydrate metabolism. Select tomato, low-salt V-8, and fresh juices from carrots or green vegetables. The nutritional profile of brown rice milk is similar to that of vegetable juices, although it does not contain any vitamin A, vitamin C, or iron. It does, however, contain vitamin E, which vegetable juices do not, and it contains the same amount of calcium.

Sodas are beverages to avoid. They are made from sugar, artificial flavors, and phosphates, which interfere with the body's calcium uptake and many contain caffeine, which affects brain function.

DAILY SERVINGS GUIDE

AGE	NUMBER OF SOY OR OTHER BEVERAGE SERVINGS
1–3 years	2
4–6 years	3
7–10 years	4
11–14 years	
girls	4
boys	5
girls 15 through adult	4
pregnant 2nd & 3rd trimesters	5
lactating	5

AGE	NUMBER OF SOY OR OTHER BEVERAGE SERVINGS
teenage boys	6
men 19 through adult	4
One beverage serving is equivalent to one cup of 2-percent cow's milk, soy, rice, or nut milks.	

CARBOHYDRATE-RICH FOODS

Carbohydrates are very important for you and your child because they supply energy for all your needs. However, the kind of carbohydrate foods you eat and what time of day you eat them can determine how they affect your brain function. I discuss the importance of carbohydrates in a previous chapter and tell why simple carbohydrates like sugar can be very detrimental to those with AD/HD. However, it is nearly impossible to eliminate all sugars from your diet. To reduce as many of them as possible, keep these simple rules in mind:

1. Never eat sugars by themselves or on an empty stomach.
2. Complex carbohydrates can calm the brain down—these are good in the evening.
3. Mixed meals of complex carbohydrates and proteins are best.
4. Eat vegetables for snacks because they contain a combination of carbohydrates and proteins, best for sustained brain function.
5. Best carbohydrate sources are whole grains, unsweetened cereals, breads, pasta, oriental noodles (rice and buckwheat, especially), and starchy vegetables.
6. When choosing breakfast cereals, read the labels carefully. If the ingredients list contains sugar or syrup anywhere, don't buy it. Usually those with sugar will contain artificial colors and preservatives as well. With this kind of cereal, you are paying a lot of money for bad ingredients.

DAILY SERVINGS GUIDE

AGE	NUMBER OF CARBOHYDRATE SERVINGS
1–3 years	4
4–6 years	6

AGE	NUMBER OF CARBOHYDRATE SERVINGS
7–10 years	7
11–14 years	
girls	7
boys	8
girls 15 through adult	7
pregnant 2nd & 3rd trimesters	8
lactating	9
teenage boys	12
men 19 through adult	13

A single serving of complex carbohydrates equals one-half cup of cereal, rice, pasta, bulgur, grits, starchy vegetables, or one slice of bread. One-third cup of lentils or beans makes up a serving.

SUGARS

There are many different kinds of sugars, and many names for them appear on labels. You should look for and avoid sugar, sucrose, fructose, dextrose, maltodextrin, brown sugar, corn or cane syrup, and high-fructose corn syrup. These are all highly refined sugars. Some sugars may be labeled natural, and these include honey, molasses, date sugar, maple sugar crystals, and fruit sweetener. They may be less processed, but they are still sugars. You should limit as much as possible the amount of *all* sugars you and, especially, your child consume. Some recipes I am providing will use maple syrup, molasses, honey, brown rice syrup, or fruit sweeteners. However, when you buy these items as separate ingredients, they are less processed, and it is easier to control how much you are using. Most of them are much sweeter than sugar. Typically, you will need only half as much.

THE GLYCEMIC INDEX

The glycemic index rates foods by how quickly they yield glucose. Foods that deliver glucose quickly have been assigned high numbers, while those that deliver glucose more slowly have been assigned lower numbers. All carbohydrate-rich foods potentially yield sugars when your body digests them. How fast they are broken into glucose, or blood sugar, depends on how complex they are. For example, when pure glucose (dextrose), a very simple sugar, is eaten, it will enter the bloodstream when it reaches the digestive system. Therefore, glucose has been assigned a value of 100 (100 percent). On the other hand, a complex carbohydrate like oatmeal will be converted slowly into glucose, which then enters the bloodstream at a much slower rate.

Why is the glycemic rate and the information it provides important to you and your AD/HD child? Eating sugary foods is not the only way to get too much sugar. Paying attention to how a food rates on the glycemic index will help you balance out the level at which sugar is entering your system. This is important as you try to balance its flow during the day. It is a matter of balance that will become more comfortable as you work with it.

GLYCEMIC INDEX

FOOD	RATING
Glucose (dextrose)	100
Carrots	92
Honey	87
Molasses	85
Brown Rice Syrup	80
Whole Wheat Bread	72
Brown Rice	66
Sucrose (table sugar)	59
Spaghetti	50
Oatmeal	49
Whole Wheat or Rice Spaghetti	42
Oranges	40
Yogurt & Ice Cream	36
Maltodextrin (pentasaccharides)	25–30
Fructose	20
Soy Beans	15
Peanuts	13
Water	0

Adapted from David Jenkins, Thomas Wolever, et al., "Glycemic Index of Foods: Physiological Bases for Carbohydrate Exchange," *American Journal of Clinical Nutrition* 34(1988):362–66.

FRUITS

Fruits contain carbohydrates and fiber but have no protein or fats. They are an excellent source of vitamins and minerals. Try to rotate the fruit you and your child eat to include as much variety as possible. Children love papayas, mangoes, pineapples, berries, melons, cherries, and kiwifruit. Often all they get are bananas, oranges, apples, and sometimes grapes.

Organically grown fruit is the best choice because it has not been gassed, sprayed, or fertilized with chemicals. You may occasionally notice small blemishes on the skin of organic fruit, but they aren't harmful. Just make sure you check the fruit as you would any fruit and remove bruises and bad spots. Because they have not been waxed, organic apples will probably not have the highly polished appeal of commercial apples. However, a vigorous rub on a towel will bring out the natural shine of a good apple. Do wash your organic fruit and vegetables to remove any lingering soil from the field. Peel any fruit that is not organic to avoid pesticides that are in the skin. If this is impractical, you should at least wash nonorganic fruit thoroughly with a food-safe soap, like Dr. Bronner's, to remove as much harmful residue as possible.

DAILY SERVINGS GUIDE

AGE	NUMBER OF FRUIT SERVINGS
1–3 years	2
4–6 years	2
7–10 years	4
11–14 years	
girls	4
boys	5
girls 15 through adult	4
pregnant 2nd & 3rd trimesters	5
lactating	6
teenage boys	6
men 19 through adult	6

Each serving is equal to one small fruit, one-half cup of cut-up fresh fruit or berries, one-quarter cup of dried fruit, or one-half cup of fruit juice.

PROTEINS

We think of protein foods, usually meat, fish, poultry, and eggs, primarily as building blocks for growth and development. Furthermore, proteins provide the essential tools for communication between brain cells, making them especially important in diets of people with AD/HD. However, this is another stumbling block you may face. Researchers have found that many AD/HD children have poor protein-digesting capability. Most often this is linked to food intolerance. Allergies can reduce digestive efficiency and the size of protein molecules entering the bloodstream. Normally, proteins are digested into smaller units called peptides and free amino acids before they can pass through the intestine. Small peptides cause no problems, but larger, undigested ones passing into the bloodstream are challenged by an individual's immune system, which causes an allergic response. Thus, a cycle is established: allergies reducing the digestion of proteins, which then pass into the bloodstream and cause further allergies.

When this happens, the brain is deprived of the necessary amino acids it needs to form its chemical messengers or neurotransmitters. Thus the allergic response also has a direct impact on brain function, leading to sluggish or inefficient mental processing.

I am approaching this problem three ways in my *30-Day Program*. We are eliminating the most common food allergens from, increasing the amount and quality of protein, and adding a good protein digestant to help the body recoup it's ability to process food effectively.

Dietary sources of concentrated proteins are fish, poultry, meat, eggs, cheese, and tofu. Beyond these sources of protein, you and your child will be getting other good sources of protein when you follow my dietary plan, such as vegetables, beans, lentils, and split peas. Grains and starchy vegetables also contain protein, but they have three times the carbohydrate content of leafy green vegetables. I have included all of these in the *30-Day Plan*. I do not recommend strict vegetarian diets for children because it is difficult to balance their proteins and they need the longer-chain polyunsaturated fatty acids found in fish. You can certainly restrict beef and veal in your child's diet if you choose. I suggest you serve lamb as much as possible when you want to eat red meat. Although lamb is not as lean as beef round, tenderloin, or sirloin, very few people are allergic to lamb, and it has been a popular substitution meat in elimination diets. Pork tenderloin is also lean and a good choice.

DAILY SERVINGS GUIDE

AGE	NUMBER OF PROTEIN SERVINGS
1–3 years	3
4–6 years	4
7–10 years	5
11–14 years	
girls	6
boys	6
girls 15 through adult	6
pregnant 2nd & 3rd trimesters	6
lactating	8
teenage boys	7
men 19 through adult	8

One serving is equal to one ounce of *less lean* cuts of beef such as steak, ground beef, roast beef, and meat loaf; one ounce of lamb, poultry, or mozzarella cheese; one-quarter cup of ricotta cheese; one egg; or four ounces of tofu. If you are planning one of these less lean proteins in your daily menu, *cut back one fat serving* that day.

High-fat proteins should be eaten infrequently, but if you are planning a dinner of barbecued ribs, sausage, hamburgers, corned beef, or prime rib, simply *eliminate most of your other fat servings that day.*

Why Diet Is Not Enough

Although a cornerstone of a lifetime of freedom from the symptoms, dietary change alone will not be sufficient to overcome AD/HD. Supplements are also essential. We have seen how AD/HD is aggravated by eating the wrong foods, and that the time of day when carbohydrates are eaten affects mental processing. Consumption of the additive-laden and highly processed foods we often eat causes irregularities in brain function that result in lack of focus, inattention, impulsivity, and hyperactivity. Now let's turn our attention to the essential micronutrients—vitamins, minerals, and fatty acids—that are also key to beating AD/HD and that you most likely are not receiving from the foods you eat.

Micronutrients determine how brain cells utilize amino acids from proteins, and glucose from carbohydrates and fats. It has taken a long time to identify which of these micronutrients are deficient in AD/HD sufferers. But, finally we have the strong scientific evidence we need to support my specific recommendations for AD/HD therapy using dietary supplements.

There are three groups of micronutrients that regulate communication between brain cells.

BRAIN – NUTRIENT CONNECTION

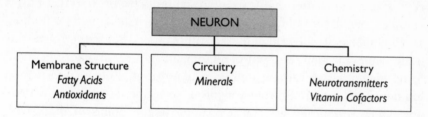

1. *Fatty acids* make up the membrane infrastructure of brain cells, they are imbedded with *antioxidants* that protect the message content and transmission apparatus.
2. *Minerals* provide for electric circuitry and fluid balance within brain cells and along nerve axons.
3. *Vitamin coenzymes* regulate the sending, receiving, and processing of messages.

Of these three groups of nutrients, the most heavily researched are the fatty acids and that's where I'll begin.

FATTY ACIDS AND BRAIN CELLS

Composed of 60 percent fats, the brain is a very fatty tissue. Most of this fatty tissue is found in the membranes that envelop neurons. The fats are highly specialized fatty acids and *phospholipids*, phosphorus-containing fatty materials. Together these fatty substances form a meshlike membrane structure that supports the tools of communication between neurons. Included in this apparatus are also proteins that function as antennae, voltage channels containing calcium and other minerals, and a layer of insulation that shoots messages down the axon. All of these devices must be exactly placed within the brain membrane for neurons to function properly. Sending and receiving signals, as well as firing instructions to brain processing centers, demand correct alignment. Those with AD/HD have disordered communication. A growing body of experts believe that the reason is that these devices are skewed, pushed out of alignment by the wrong dietary fats and specific micronutrient deficiencies.

The brain is made up of 100 billion neurons and it contains more active surface area than any other organ in your body. That's a lot of surface structure to have malfunction. No wonder AD/HD occurs when brain cells cannot communicate! Dietary modification and supplements to reconfigure neuronal membranes are indispensable to relieving the confusing mind chatter that is so often symptomatic of AD/HD. This is because your brain is highly selective in which fats it prefers. If those aren't available, it will grudgingly substitute others, but the surrogate fats push communication tools out of alignment. As a result, your attention, focus, memory, and learning ability are all impaired. Enough information has now been gathered through vigorous scientific investigation that we now know specifically what is happening in the brains of those with AD/HD.

Several studies have compared fatty acid levels in AD/HD children with those of normal children. Researchers have confirmed that lower levels of the critical fatty acids exist in the red blood cells and serum of AD/HD individuals. Supplementing AD/HD sufferers' diets with the correct fatty acids has reversed their hyperactivity, aggression, and impulsiveness. What are these fats, where do they come from, and how can they overcome AD/HD?

LCPs: The Correct Fatty Acids

We tend to think all fats are bad, but some are essential—you must get them from your diet. Two families of essential fats, the *omega-6 fatty acids* and the *omega-3 fatty acids* come from dietary sources. Omega-6 (cis-linoleic acid) comes from soy and canola oils, and omega-3 (alpha-linolenic acid) from flaxseed (linseed) oil. Linoleic and linolenic fatty acids are nutritionally important because they are precursors of the long-chain polyunsaturated fatty acids (LCPs) needed by our brain cells.

Dietary Essential Fatty Acids or EFAs are of two types

Omega-6 or n-6 from linoleic acid (canola, olive, safflower, and corn oils)
Omega-3 or n-3 from alpha-linolenic acid (flaxseed oil)

Dietary EFAs have to be converted into long-chain polyunsaturated fatty acids (LCPs)

Omega-6: gamma-linolenic acid (GLA), dihomo-gamma-linolenic acid (DGLA), and arachidonic acid (AA)
Omega-3: eicosapentaenoic acid (EPA) and docosahexaenoic acid (DHA)

Our changing dietary practices in the last hundred years, especially the last half of this century, have unbalanced the natural ratios in our bodies between omega-6 and omega-3 fatty acids. The reduction of natural resources like fish, game, and homegrown produce, in favor of feedlot-raised beef, mass-produced poultry, farm-raised fish, and widespread alteration of foods, has greatly reduced our intake of these fatty acids. That's why eating the wrong kind of animal (or vegetable) fats is a major contributor to symptoms of AD/HD and most other chronic conditions we battle today. This is especially true in small children, who are not efficient at making LCPs. High-carbohydrate diets and carbohydrate-related disorders interfere with the body's ability to manufacture LCPs. Other factors that can block these enzymes are environmental stress, alcohol or prescription drug use, viral infections, natural aging, and deficiencies of vitamins and minerals.

Although we can synthesize LCPs from our diet, we have evolved over the centuries with diets so rich in these, we have little need to manufacture our own. In September 1998, Michael Crawford, an eminent researcher from England, presented evidence confirming this fact at a conference on fatty acids sponsored by the National Institutes of Mental Health. Dr. Crawford pointed out that the ratios between omega-3 and omega-6 fatty acids have gradually changed from 1:1 to 1:30 as we have eaten more cultivated and less wild game and ocean source foods. These changes have been most pronounced in the last 200 years. Our hunter-gatherer ancestors obtained plenty of these fatty acids directly from their food, hence the enzymatic conversion from seed oils into LCPs was not developed to the degree today's lifestyle demands. These enzymes are *metabolic enzymes*, a group distinct from digestive enzymes, and they are very sensitive to recent changes in our diet and lifestyle.

The enzymes, *delta-5 desaturase* and *delta-6 desaturase*, transform linoleic acid, linoleates, and linolenates into LCPs. They are easily baffled by the wrong kind of dietary fats, such as those that are saturated or hydrogenated. These same two enzymes convert both families of fatty acids into LCPs, but they do not cross family lines. In other words, when a deficiency of an omega-3 fatty acid occurs, the enzymes cannot substitute omega-6 fatty acids to make up the deficit. The LCPs we are concerned with are docosahexaenoic (DHA), arachidonic (AA), and gamma-linolenic (GLA). The only one of these that is an omega-3 is DHA.

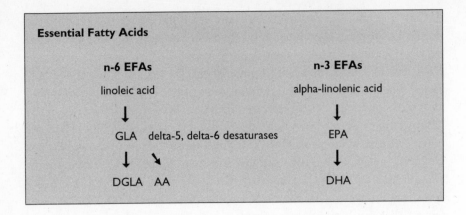

WHY LCP SUPPLEMENTS ARE NEEDED

If our LCP levels are now, we can get them directly from our diet. That means eating good animal and vegetable sources of LCPs or taking dietary supplements that provide them. Strict vegetarian (vegan) diets contain plenty of linoleic and linolenic fatty acids that are the direct predecessors of LCPs. Yet, those on vegan diets are usually low in LCPs because of their bodies' inefficient processing of the fatty acids in dietary oils. The high-carbohydrate diet of vegetarians may also reduce LCP conversion. I do not recommend vegetarian or low-fat diets for children, especially those with AD/HD, because of these conditions. Let's see how AD/HD-related conditions result from low levels of specific LCPs.

LCP DEFICIENCIES AND ALLERGIES

Allergies disrupt fatty acid metabolism, and common symptoms among children are dry skin and hair, excessive thirst, and frequency of urination. Allergies and food sensitivities can also cause behavioral problems—including AD/HD, as we have seen. Not surprisingly, there is a connection here. It was the high incidence of allergies in AD/HD individuals that gave scientists their first clue to what might be missing in the diets of AD/HD individuals. LCP deficiencies were found to be the common ground between these disorders. When scientists pursued this discovery, they solved a large piece of the puzzle that is ADD.

Today, we get only about half the amount of LCPs from animal sources as we did fifty years ago. Not only have we come to rely less upon wild game and ocean source foods as years have passed, but we also have changed the way we feed animals from free ranging to corn- and grain-fed. This is true of cattle, hogs, poultry, and farm-grown fish. Both of these changes have decreased the LCPs we take in. A pregnant woman usually depends heavily on dairy products for calcium and other important nutrients, including LCPs, needed for her unborn child to develop a healthy brain and body. If a woman doesn't get adequate dietary levels of LCPs, each successive pregnancy will deplete her of them even further. Today we are faced with generations of children malnourished by these LCP-deficient diets. And lack of these fatty acids is a major reason we have so many children diagnosed today with AD/HD. If we don't address AD/HD nutritionally, this situation can only get worse.

LCPs BEFORE BIRTH

It has been known for some time that LCPs are critical to the developing embryo from the first weeks following conception until gestation. However, even before conception occurs, fertility problems can be traced to lack of LCPs. Activation and hormonal balance in both men and women rely on LCPs, and they are a necessary element in sperm formation. Therefore every couple contemplating parenthood should be sure to add an LCP supplement to their diets. For mothers-to-be this is especially important.

At birth, the baby has most of the neurons it will have throughout life; the fetus has absorbed whatever nutrients it needed and were available from its mother during pregnancy. Thus, a woman who has marginal LCP status either at the beginning or during pregnancy will show extremely low LCP levels when her baby is born. If she has this deficiency, she will likely suffer from postpartum depression as well, which is considered a symptom of this nutritional deficit. It has been estimated that 70 percent of American women today suffer "baby blues," and one in five hundred will go on to develop major depression. This is precisely what happened to Ann, Justin and Jennifer's mother.

Women who do not restore healthy levels of LCPs after a child is born and before becoming pregnant again run an even greater risk of having an AD/HD child. Just think how many lives could be changed with this information! If you are considering pregnancy, or know someone who is, tell them about LCPs. It makes sense to add them to every pre-pregnancy and prenatal nutrition program because many women are already marginally deficient when they become pregnant.

All three LCPs are strongly linked to successful pregnancy and normal birth weight. GLA is important to development of a healthy placenta to filter and nourish the infant while in utero. AA is associated with normal birth weight, circumference of the baby's head, placental weight, and cardiovascular development. DHA is essential to brain and nervous system maturity at birth, and it is the most plentiful fatty acid in these organs as well as the eyes and heart. There is compelling evidence that even normal-birth-weight children who later have attention deficits and other neurological disorders are undernourished at birth in at least one of these EFAs as well as important vitamins and minerals.

LCPs and the Newborn

By the time an infant is born, its body has already manufactured the 100 billion or so brain cells it will depend on throughout life. Some new neurons will develop until the infant reaches eighteen months, but *interneuron* connections will continue to be built throughout its life. The interneuron connections allow us to add new experiences to our arsenal of information. A network of glial cells tend to the nutritional and other

INTERNEURON CONNECTIONS

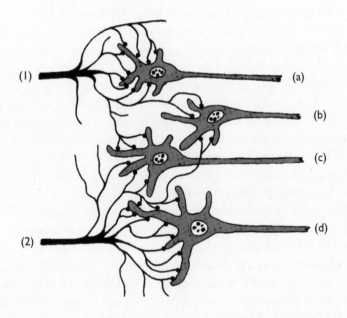

Axon (1) note the interneuron connections with (a), (b) and (c), but not (d)
Axon (2) note the interneuron connection with (b), (c) and (d), but not (a)

Neurons send instructions to areas of the brain for processing by forming interneuron connections. Only those connections needed are formed. We add new connections throughout life, as they are needed.

needs of neurons. All of these brain structures rely on LCPs. That's why even children and adults without any apparent symptoms of AD/HD or other neuro-impairments can benefit from supplements of LCPs as well. We can always improve brain nutrition. According to Professor Michael Crawford of the Institute of Brain Chemistry and Human Nutrition, University of North London, England, "the deficits with AA and DHA at birth must surely signal much wider nutritional deficits which are unlikely to be confined to fatty acids." This is why my recommendations for nutritional correction of AD/HD include vitamins and minerals as well as fatty acids.

Many AD/HD individuals are sensitive to bright light and have impaired night vision because their ability to adjust to either bright or dim light is reduced. LCPs are an integral part of the visual apparatus, especially the rod photoreceptors, which distinguish action in dim light. There are a total of 125 million photoreceptors in the retina of each eye. It is amazing how much membrane surface the eye has, a property it shares with the brain, and both are composed primarily of excitable nervous tissues that rely on LCPs to function.

The newborn comes equipped with a complete visual apparatus, but because his eyes have not been exposed to light, vision cannot be fully developed until after birth. The millions of photoreceptors transfer information they receive to the visual cortex of the brain, a process that takes a mere thousandth of a second. If they are low in LCPs, the process is thwarted, just as in the brain, and visual response is reduced as a result. Nature has carefully provided for the exceptionally high LCP demand of the infant brain and eyes with the perfect food—mother's milk.

FUNCTIONS OF LCPs IN INFANTS

Human breast milk contains very high levels of LCPs, especially DHA and AA. Breast milk ensures the infant will have levels of DHA needed for brain and eye development. Unfortunately, infant formula manufacturers in the United States and Canada do not fortify their products with DHA or AA. It seems that feeding a baby breast milk rather than formula could therefore make a difference in the baby's brain function. There is evidence to back up this hypothesis.

Several studies, among them one by A. Lucas and colleagues in 1992 and another by Maria Makrides in 1995, have measured differences in intelligence quotient between children who were bottle-fed and those who were breast-fed. The latter appear to have a measurable I.Q. advantage, perhaps stemming from their higher LCP intake.

As for vision, in 1992 Eileen Birch and her group from the Retina Foundation in Dallas studied the importance of DHA in visual development. They found improved vision in breast-fed infants over formula-fed infants and reported their findings in the *Journal of Pediatric Ophthalmology & Strabismus*. Once bottle-fed infants were supplemented with LCPs, they enjoyed the same benefits as their breast-fed counterparts. But, there are further advantages beyond improved intelligence and enhanced vision for breast-fed babies.

In January of 1998, a study was published in the *British Medical Journal* by A. C. Wilson and colleagues that examined whether breast-feeding had long-term effects on respiratory illnesses, growth, body mass index, percentage of body fat, and blood pressure. The study was a seven-year follow-up of 545 children who had been exclusively fed breast milk for the first fifteen weeks of life. The scientists concluded that the incidence of respiratory illness occurring at any time during childhood was considerably reduced by breast-feeding. This study confirms what most parents believe about breast-feeding—that it affords better resistance to infection—and why they opt for this feeding method despite the inconvenience for working mothers. Are LCPs the ingredient in breast milk that provides immunity?

LCPs are not the only substances needed to build immunity, but they are a major factor, since low levels are strongly correlated with increased frequency of infections. An earlier study at Purdue University found that children who had adequate blood levels of LCPs experienced significantly fewer infections and antibiotic use. Breast milk, but not formula, provides these LCPs, and that at least partially accounts for the higher resistance to illness seen in breast-fed babies.

LCP SUPPLEMENTS FOR PREGNANCY AND LACTATION

Breast-feeding among American women confers obvious advantages to their babies, and that's in spite of the fact that American women have one of the lowest levels of LCPs in breast milk in the world. The typical American diet is wreaking havoc with our children, beginning in pregnancy and continuing during lactation and throughout the growth of years. We can halt the negative impact of our nutritional deficiencies on their health by supplementing the diet of both pregnant and lactating women with LCPs and other nutrients I discuss. Just as we have found that women of childbearing age should take folic acid to prevent neural tube defects, LCP supplementation should be an accepted part of prenatal and lactating nutrition programs. What about babies fed formula—what can we do for them?

LCP FORTIFICATION OR SUPPLEMENTATION FOR INFANT FORMULAS

Manufacturers in the United States and Canada add linoleic acid to their infant formulas, but it doesn't benefit infants who do not have the capability to transform it into LCPs. Effects of low levels of LCPs are most pronounced in premature and low-birth-weight infants. Sheila Innis, from the Department of Pediatrics at the University of British Columbia, has found that bottle-fed infants consistently have low levels of AA and DHA in their blood serum and red blood cells, even those born full-term. Her findings were reported in the *Journal of Pediatrics* in 1992.

Here we are seven years later, and we still don't have LCP fortification of infant formula despite widespread fortification in many other countries. DHA fortification has been strongly recommended here in the United States and around the world by the World Health Organization and the Food and Agriculture Organization. I hope baby formula in the United States soon contains this important nutrient. In the meantime, you can add a DHA supplement directly to your baby's bottle once a day. I will tell you the appropriate amount to add in the supplement chapter.

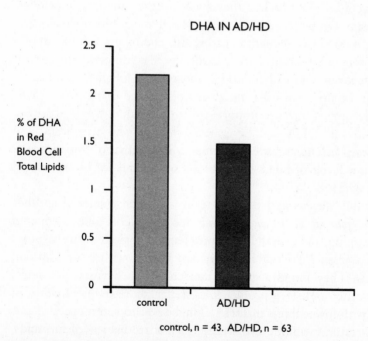

DHA IN AD/HD

% of DHA in Red Blood Cell Total Lipids

control, n = 43. AD/HD, n = 63

Stevens et al., *American Journal of Clinical Nutrition* 62 (1995): 761.

HOW DO DHA AND AA AFFECT BRAIN FUNCTION?

Let's move on to older children and see if those with AD/HD have lower LCP levels than their non-AD/HD counterparts. Laura Stevens and John Burgess of Purdue University published results in the *American Journal of Clinical Nutrition* of a 1994 study on DHA levels in fifty-three boys with clinically diagnosed AD/HD. The AD/HD boys had significantly lower levels of DHA than did the forty-three boys who did not have AD/HD. This study and that of Dr. Innis have shown us a new way to approach the treatment of AD/HD.

DHA is the primary fatty acid in neurons, making up 30 percent of our total brain fat content. It is produced in us and other animals through a series of enzymatic steps from alpha-linolenic acid, found in seed oils, primarily linseed (flax). It is also in certain kinds of highly nutritive micro-algae that are a large part of the diets of fish and marine mammals, particularly those of the deep, cold waters of the north Atlantic and northern Pacific oceans.

We have known for some time about the health benefits of eating deep cold-water fish, primarily because of the heart-friendly EPAs that they contain. EPAs reduce platelet stickiness, a major contributor to stroke and heart attack. Platelets are tiny blood cells that contain clotting factors needed to stem bleeding. When they stick together, the fragile platelets break, releasing the factors and forming clots that can block arteries and impede blood flow. Consequently, eating fish and taking fish oil supplements has been an important part of cardiovascular protection programs.

Little attention was paid to DHA, the other LCP in the omega-3 family, until recently. But it has now been discovered that DHA is plentiful in body organs that are impulse-driven, including the heart, eyes, brain, and nerves. DHA maintains heart rhythm, and eye, brain, and nerve function. Scientists have confirmed a link between visual impairments and low levels of DHA in the blood serum and red blood cells of those with AD/HD.

In 1995, the Stevens and Burgess team published results of another trial in the *Journal of Physiology and Behavior*. This one compared behavior, learning, and overall health problems in boys six to twelve years old who had *lowered levels of both fatty acid families* with boys who had higher levels. They found a greater incidence of behavioral problems, temper tantrums, and sleep problems, as well as more frequent colds, in those boys with lower levels of DHA. The boys who had more frequent colds and greater antibiotic use were also low in omega-6 fatty acids, including GLA and its immune-boosting, inflammation-fighting product, dihomo-gamma-linolenic acid (DGLA). GLA and DGLA also correct hormone imbalances.

LCP Supplementation for Related Disorders

A deficiency of one LCP generally indicates that others are deficient as well. Specific indications of GLA deficiency are frequent infections; dry skin, scalp, and hair; extreme thirstiness; need to urinate frequently; hormone imbalances; and PMS. There is a vast body of information on DHA deficiencies resulting in neuropsychological disorders including AD/HD and vision problems and on GLA deficiencies in skin and immune disorders. Therefore it is a good idea to take both DHA and GLA supplements. Diets may supply enough AA for older children and adults, but infant diets should be supplemented with this fatty acid as well. The supplement recommendations I will make provide for these fatty acids.

Now that we've settled the issue of membrane structure and function, let's see what is needed to improve the action of brain cells.

Minerals and Brain Circuitry

In the mid-seventies, just at the time Dr. Feingold was gaining fame and notoriety for his concepts, my mind was opened by the wisdom of another physician. His name was Carl Pfeiffer and he was director and founder of the Brain-Bio Center in Princeton, New Jersey. Even back then, Dr. Pfeiffer believed that AD/HD, called minimal brain dysfunction at the time, could be alleviated by correcting brain chemistry through diet and appropriate supplementation. Not many people were espousing such ideas.

What most impressed me about Dr. Pfeiffer's work was his introduction of the importance of mineral balance in the brain. What is so interesting about how vitamins and minerals act in the brain is the high degree of interaction between them. Perhaps this is what has boggled scientists for so long. The foundation of our modern scientific method is to test isolated substances for their effects, yet it is almost impossible to do this with nutrients. However, there have been a few good studies on the way in which individual nutrients act on brain function.

The earth provides us with ninety-two naturally occurring elements. Most of them are metals or minerals. Some are gases, like hydrogen, oxygen, and nitrogen. We need some of them for various bodily functions, but as we saw in earlier chapters, we get too much of many. Now, I'm going to tell you about those the brain needs and often has trouble getting.

CALCIUM, MAGNESIUM, AND AD/HD

Brain function depends on a few key minerals that make up only 0.5 percent of the brain's weight. Whereas fatty acids provide much of the bulk of the brain, minerals constitute a small fraction of its mass. Even so, they are a crucial ingredient in healthy brain function that insure the activation of neuronal communication, regulation of brain metabolism, and protection of the brain against free-radical oxidation and toxic-metal contamination. Calcium and magnesium have the biggest role in brain function and make up most of the mineral content in the brain.

Calcium is a second messenger in neuronal membranes, which means it acts like a traffic signal for uptake and release of neurotransmitters. A "green light" from calcium permits release of a neurotransmitter into the synaptic intersection, and a "red light" halts its passage into the receiving neuron. Calcium also interacts with potassium and sodium to maintain proper levels of nerve-cell stimulation, and this is how balance between nerve activation and inactivation is achieved in the brain. In addition, calcium interacts with zinc in the regulation of the neurotransmitter histamine and is dependent on DHA for all of its membrane functions. Thus, calcium regulates the speed, intensity, and clarity of every message that passes between brain cells. Most people have no idea calcium is so important in regulating the brain.

Unfortunately, the USDA reports that 30 percent of Americans, including children, are low in calcium, magnesium, zinc, and other trace minerals. In order to correct errors in neurotransmission, we must increase our intake of these minerals. Paradoxically, these three minerals compete for uptake into our systems, increasing the difficulty of introducing a sufficient amount of each of them into our diet. This makes the form in which we supplement them for AD/HD extremely important. I will discuss how minerals should be purchased in Part IV.

Now, let's look at magnesium and its effects on AD/HD.

In 1997, a Polish research team headed by Tadeusz Kozielec assessed magnesium levels in 116 children with AD/HD. Ninety-seven of the nine- to twelve-year-old children were boys, and twenty were girls. Sixty-eight of them (fifty boys, eighteen girls) had other disorders such as enuresis, tics, stuttering, and separation anxiety coexisting with AD/HD. As we have seen, these conditions are typical in a population of AD/HD children. The scientists found low magnesium levels in 95 percent of the children regardless of whether they had coexisting conditions.

Subsequently, the researchers began magnesium supplementation with seventy-five of the magnesium-deficient AD/HD children with coexisting conditions. In addition, all of the children were receiving anti-psychotic or other nonstimulant therapy for AD/HD. Fifty of the children received six milligrams of magnesium per pound (6 mg/lb) of body weight for six months, and the remaining twenty-five served as controls. The supplemented children showed a magnesium increase in body tissues and a decrease in hyperactivity. The control children remained the same. This leads us to believe just how profound the effects on behavior can be if just one mineral imbalance is reversed in AD/HD children.

Zinc is the third most important mineral in the brain. Most zinc is concentrated in the brain membranes, where it acts like an antioxidant to protect DHA, AA, and the phospholipids from free-radical attack. However, zinc also acts on the surface of neurons as an electrical "contact" for neurotransmission, and it helps convert serotonin (5-hydroxytryptamine or 5-HTP) into melatonin, which is an important regulator of biorhythms.

Two important studies were completed in 1996 that checked zinc status in AD/HD children. The first was done in Israel, and the second was done in Poland. Dr. Paz Toren and colleagues at the Tel-Aviv Community Health Center tested blood serum zinc levels from forty-three children aged six to sixteen, most of whom were male. They matched the ages of the AD/HD group with twenty-eight normal children who served as controls. They found serum zinc levels were significantly lower in the AD/HD group, averaging two-thirds the levels of those without AD/HD.

The research team noted that the children were generally well nourished and ate a balanced diet. It was noted, however, that AD/HD children are often picky eaters and it is difficult to get them to sit down and eat a decent meal. This is yet another insight as to why dietary supplements are so important in overcoming AD/HD.

Professors Sidney V. Stohs and Debasis Bagchi, of Creighton University in Omaha, Nebraska, contributed to the information on zinc's role by examining the previous work that had been done on zinc's antioxidant function. From the accumulated evidence, they concluded that zinc displaces other minerals that have demonstrated free-radical potential. Iron and copper are two such minerals. They described the protection of LCPs from free-radical damage as either "push" or "pull" actions. Zinc pushes the potentially harmful minerals out of the way. In comparison, vitamin C and related cofactors pull possibly harmful metals aside by "chelating" them.

VITAMIN C AND ITS COFACTORS IN BRAIN FUNCTION

The brain contains more vitamin C than any other body organ with the exception of the adrenal glands. Vitamin C is necessary to the body's manufacture of norepinephrine, dopamine, and serotonin, three of the neurotransmitters involved in AD/HD. It is also required if the body is to utilize folic acid, which is another vitamin needed for normal development of the central nervous system.

Vitamin C also protects the brain from free-radical damage induced by iron, copper, heavy metals, environmental toxins, or oxygen free radicals. One of the most remarkable protections vitamin C affords is the chelation of reactive metals such as lead, mercury, cadmium, and aluminum. Chelation "wraps up" the metal so it can be eliminated from the body.

The effects of vitamin C are enhanced by its cofactors, known as flavan-3-ols, and these also protect vitamin C so that it isn't destroyed. These factors, also called *proanthocyanidins*, are members of a large class of protective phenolic compounds that we get from fruits and vegetables. They have been the subject of numerous scientific investigations and their efficacy has been validated by scientists throughout the world. Available in Europe for nearly forty years as prescription drugs for the treatment of venous conditions, these compounds have the unique property of strengthening the walls of arteries, veins, and capillaries, including brain microcapillaries. Oligomeric proanthocyanidins (OPCs), marketed either as Masquelier's OPCs or Pycnogenol, appear to have a number of other properties that explain their benefits to AD/HD.

BLOCKING HISTAMINE TO REDUCE INFLAMMATION AND SWELLING

Allergies are rampant among those with AD/HD, and they cause histamine release that increases fluid around brain cells. As we have seen, the brain gets "waterlogged" from the excess fluid, and function becomes impaired. Masquelier's OPCs, a trade name for the original pine bark and grape seed extract products developed by Dr. Jacques Masquelier in the 1940s, block histamine and can be thought of as "nature's antihistamines." They also block inflammation by moderating the production of pro-inflammatory agents produced from AA that escapes from its membrane-bound position.

These remarkable flavanols protect vitamin C and enhance its numerous antioxidant and coenzyme effects, especially in the brain and eyes. These, and antihistamine, anti-inflammatory, and immune-boosting effects, make OPCs an essential part of my *30-Day Plan*, but that's not all they do! OPCs affect the metabolic enzymes that regulate neurotransmitters in ways that are not entirely clear and are now being studied extensively. They readily pass the blood brain barrier, and a number of in-vitro studies have shown them to protect against many substances that can harm the brain in the developing fetus. They have also been shown to inhibit breakdown of the catecholamine neurotransmitters, norepinephrine and dopamine, and moderate the activity of cellular enzymes, which improves the processing of information. These are no doubt some of the major ways by which they have been found to increase attention and reduce hyperactivity.

THE EVIDENCE FOR AD/HD

Clinical evidence of the effectiveness of OPCs had come from many sources. One is a psychiatric team in Tulsa, Oklahoma, who found twenty-seven adults and children with AD/HD scored as well when they were taking Masquelier's OPC as they previously had when taking stimulant medication. Marian Sigurdson, Ph.D., directed the trial in a Tulsa medical clinic. The team found that administration of OPCs reduced hyperactivity and increased attention and focus as effectively as Ritalin.

James Greenblatt, M.D., a child psychiatrist in Boston, Massachusetts, has reported success in reducing AD/HD symptoms with OPCs as well. Dr. Greenblatt employs EEG biofeedback to measure his patients' responsiveness to therapies he uses. With such tools, Dr. Greenblatt found that OPCs reduced the number of theta waves—the daydreaming state—in his young AD/HD patients so that their attention was significantly increased.

TRACE MINERALS AND AD/HD

Iron, manganese, copper, cobalt, and molybdenum regulate brain metabolism by activating the metabolic enzymes. We are aware of selenium's protective role throughout the body, but there have not been many investigations of its effects on brain protection. However, in a 1995 study at Istanbul's Medical University, selenium was shown to protect the integrity of message sending between neurons by preventing free-radical attack. Chromium regulates glucose uptake and metabolism, and thus is vital in assuming sufficient energy for brain activities. Unfortunately, it is another element researchers believe might be deficient in the U.S. population.

According to a U.S. Department of Health, Education, and Welfare report issued in 1979, American children are very low in trace minerals. This doesn't surprise leading nutritional scientists like Lindsay Allen, Ph.D., from the University of California at Davis. According to Dr. Allen, children don't have just one micronutrient deficiency. If iron or any other trace mineral is low, the others will be as well. Poor iron status among U.S. children is of particular concern because of the number of our children who have AD/HD. It has been estimated from recent surveys that 8 percent of those children four years and under are low in iron, 13 percent of those aged five to twelve, and another 8 percent of fifteen- to forty-nine-year-olds are deficient in iron. For many years, experts have warned that children who are low in iron are at risk for mental disorders, even mental retardation in the most severe cases. I recommend that you have blood cell levels of all the trace minerals tested in yourself and your children if you suspect you are suffering from AD/HD.

Dr. Allen has worked for many years with world organizations to improve micronutrient status among children. Iron status has been one of her major concerns, because she has seen that food fortification with iron is not effective. She and her colleagues at Davis have determined Ferrochel, an amino acid chelated iron, was most effective as a supplement. Ferrochel is highly bioavailable and not affected by food phytates, which bind iron so that it cannot be utilized. I suggest you try to find and supplement with Ferrochel if you discover a deficiency of iron in you or your AD/HD child.

B VITAMINS AND AD/HD

Of the B-vitamin group, vitamin B_6 (pyridoxine) has been the most studied in brain disorders although it is not the only important B vitamin. Researchers have found that vitamin B_6 levels can be depressed by many agents, including environmental toxins. According to a report by A. L. Bernstein, published in the *Annals of the New York Academy of Science*, many conditions in clinical neurology can be improved with a vitamin B_6 supplement. Among them are seizures, autism, depression, headaches, and chronic pain, many of which are often associated with AD/HD. It is important to be aware of this and take vitamin B_6 to keep your levels up if you are facing AD/HD.

Faulty neurotransmission is considered the leading reason for inattention, hyperactivity, impulsivity, temper tantrums, sleep disorders, forgetfulness, and aggression. As we have seen, four neurotransmitters are involved. Dopamine and norepinephrine are thought to control attention and hyperactivity. Serotonin, or 5-hydroxytryptamine (5-HTP), appears to regulate depression, aggression, sleep, pain, impulsivity, and eating disorders. The neurotransmitter acetylcholine plays an important role in memory. All of these neurotransmitters are synthesized in the brain from dietary precursors. In order for this to occur, vitamin B_6, magnesium, zinc, ascorbate, biotin, folic acid, and niacin all must be present. Given the symptoms of deficiency, it is not much of a surprise that behavioral disorders including AD/HD respond well to supplementation with these nutrients. The need for supplementation in AD/HD sufferers may be due to several factors, including inadequate dietary sources, inability to extract needed amounts, or because they require more than others.

In a study conducted in England in the late 1970s, Mary Coleman, Ph.D., and colleagues found hyperkinetic children had 50 percent lower blood levels of serotonin than nonhyperactive children. The research team knew that vitamin B_6 (pyridoxine) elevates serotonin levels, and they wanted to know if vitamin B_6 was just as effective as methylphenidate in alleviating hyperactivity.

The six children in the trial (five boys, one girl) were taking methylphenidate. During the twenty-one-day trial, the children alternated between taking a placebo and high and low doses of both methylphenidate and pyridoxine. Behavior-rating scales were used to assess their response. In all cases, the children had fewer behavioral infractions when taking the higher dose of pyridoxine than either dose of methylphenidate. Moreover, the teacher and parent behavioral observers noted a carryover effect during placebo administration following vitamin B_6 administration. This suggests a "repair" effect. During pyridoxine administration, blood serotonin levels were also raised. Although pyridoxine, or vitamin B_6, was the specific B vitamin tested, the other B vitamins are required to "push" pyridoxine-activated enzymatic reactions to completion.

You can see that the argument for supplementation with fatty acids, minerals, and vitamins is extremely compelling. In the early eighties, a Canadian team noted that the data accumulated proved diet alone could not provide enough nutrients to overcome fluctuation in brain biochemistry. They urged more study of the vitamins and minerals involved in the synthesis of the five neurotransmitters serotonin, the catecholamines, acetylcholine, histamine, and glycine.

One could wish others had listened to them and more time and resources had been allocated to study specific effects and optimum dosages of micronutrients needed by those with AD/HD. It seems apparent that ratios between the minerals might be tailored to suit the individual, based on his or her biochemical data. This is something you should take up with your doctor. I am providing information on this kind of testing in appendix 4. My suggestions for dietary supplementation in later chapters are based on clinical experience and the scientific data that are available. But we all must keep in mind that more research in this vein would be extremely helpful to those struggling with AD/HD and that we should do what we can to get it implemented and funded.

PART IV

The 30-Day Plan

We have an infinite amount to learn both
from nature and from each other.

—*John Glenn*

CHAPTER 14

Recommended Supplements

In previous chapters, I shared the scientific studies that have identified the dietary supplements needed to help overcome AD/HD and elaborated on the outcomes of preliminary and clinical trials that used specific supplements to alleviate AD/HD. Now, I'd like to discuss a supplement plan based on these and other research findings.

But first let me say that several of the supplements I am recommending in my *30-Day Plan* are currently undergoing full-scale clinical trials in the United States to determine their effectiveness in reducing AD/HD symptoms specifically. In some cases the supplements are being tested against stimulants, which are the accepted way to treat AD/HD. I want to mention this fact as further proof that the move toward a nutritional answer to AD/HD is being embraced on a wide scale and so you can be on the lookout for the results of these trials.

WHAT'S GOING ON IN RESEARCH TODAY

• A team at Baylor University in New Orleans completed a trial in June 1998 prescribing Neuromins DHA to adolescent students who had previously been taking Ritalin. Results of this trial will be published in 1999.

- Laura Stevens and John Burgess have conducted two previous studies on the levels of essential LCPs, primarily DHA, on individuals with AD/HD. This Purdue University team completed a trial in 1998 using a composite fatty acid formula called Focus to reduce symptoms of AD/HD in children and adults. The results of this trail will also be published in 1999.
- Several other teams are studying the effects of DHA on Alzheimer's disease, cancer, male fertility, and postpartum depression. You should begin to hear the results of these studies in 1999.
- Pycnogenol is currently the subject of a trial at the Attention Deficit Center in St. Louis, Missouri. The trial is designed for adults with AD/HD because the disorder is somewhat newly recognized and appropriate protocols for adults have not been developed. The adult syndrome impacts family members, peer relationships, and careers in ways not fully understood. Currently the only therapy has been stimulant medication and/or depressants, which do not work the same way in adults with AD/HD as they do in children. The trial is a double-blind, randomized crossover trial of thirty AD/HD adults plus matched controls, and is being conducted by Steven Tenenbaum, Ph.D., and Julie Paull, Ph.D. Results from this trial will also be published in 1999.

THE 30-DAY SUPPLEMENT PLAN

I am now going to make specific recommendations on products you should purchase for your *30-Day Plan*. I have suggested specific supplements here because these are the ones that are backed by current research. Others I am recommending because, in my twenty years of using various brands, I have found they work best. In many cases, the supplement types I mention are available from several manufacturers. Just be sure to specify the specific supplement name I mention when shopping. It would be best if you do not make any substitutions here because I have carefully researched these exact items and found they have the best results in reducing AD/HD. In order to have the success your child deserves, you must follow my recommendations carefully.

OMEGA-3 FATTY ACIDS

Fatty acid products for AD/HD that have proven themselves clinically effective and have been used in controlled trials are as follows:

PRODUCT *Neuromins DHA*

This is a vegetable source of DHA cultured from a micro-algae. Neuromins products are available in several forms. The most popular are capsules containing between 100 mg and 500 mg of DHA in a safflower-oil base with vitamins C and E added as antioxidants to protect the oils. These soft gelatin capsules are free of any contaminants and have passed extremely rigid requirements for use in infant formulas. A granular form is also available.

USE FOR Supplementation during the prenatal period, lactation, and in infant formulas, to modify behavior in non-AD/HD children as well as in AD/HD children and adults. Neuromins is used preventively as well as to correct deficiencies.

HOW MUCH? Pregnant and lactating women: 200 mg per day
Infants: 100 mg per day, capsule contents squeezed into formula
Children (AD/HD): 400 mg in two divided doses
Children (non-AD/HD): 200 mg in two divided doses
Adults (AD/HD): 800 mg in two divided doses
Adults (non-AD/HD): 400 mg in two divided doses

PRODUCT *Focus*

This, a combination of tuna oil and evening primrose oil, is the second fatty acid product that has been well researched. It contains three LCPs—DHA, AA, and GLA—in a balanced ratio. Each soft gelatin capsule contains 60 mg of DHA, 12 mg of GLA, and 5 mg of AA plus 1 mg of thyme oil and vitamin E to protect the oils.

USE FOR School-age children, adolescents, and adults with AD/HD, especially if they have allergies. This formula is a good balance of the three LCPs needed for correcting deficiencies.

HOW MUCH? Children: 8 capsules daily in two divided doses
Adolescents: 8 capsules in two divided doses
Adults, mild AD/HD: 8 capsules daily in two divided doses
Adults, severe AD/HD: 12 capsules daily in three divided doses

You may have wondered why the same amounts of the products are recommended for children and adults. Since we are feeding the brain, and both children and adults have about the same number of neurons, it requires the same amount of LCPs to rewire the brain.

OMEGA-6 FATTY ACIDS

PRODUCT *Evening primrose oil*

    This is a source of GLA and its precursor cis-linoleic acid. The same conditions that impede your body's ability to convert dietary precursors into omega-3's also reduce the availability of omega-6's, namely GLA. That's one of the main reasons why infections and inflammatory conditions such as allergies are common in those with AD/HD. You will have to be very selective in the evening primrose oil you choose. Do not shop just for price. Insist on splitting open a capsule before you buy the product to see if it is rancid. Rancidity can be detected by a strong acrid odor and a stinging sensation on your tongue when you sample the oil in the capsule. A good evening primrose oil should be a clear golden color and odorless.

USE FOR Reducing allergic symptoms, incidence of infections, and lowered immune resistance. Also helpful for balancing hormone levels in teens and adults.

HOW MUCH? Children: 500 mg capsules, each containing 45 mg of GLA, 3 capsules a day with meals.
               Adults: 6 capsules per day with meals.

    When using both DHA and evening primrose oil, maintain a ratio of four parts DHA to one part GLA (4 DHA: 1 GLA). This ratio helps restore the natural balance between omega-3's and omega-6's.

VITAMIN C AND COFACTORS

PRODUCT *Masquelier's OPCs, Pycnogenol,* and *Berkem's Authentic Gold OPCs.*

    There are many grape seed extract products on the market, but these are the best. Masquelier's and Berkem's grape seed extracts are still manufactured using the same methods originated by Dr. Masquelier over forty years ago. These products have the approval of the French Ministry of Health and meet rigorous pharmaceutical standards. Pycnogenol has also been extensively researched. Like Berkem's Pinebark Gold, Pycnogenol is an extract from French Maritime Pine that has been extensively researched. I recommend you first try either Masquelier's or Berkem's grape seed OPC products because they contain higher levels of the principal actives, so you need less.

However, some people may get better results with pine-bark-extract OPCs because the overall chemical composition differs between grape seed OPC and pine bark OPC. Many active compounds are found in these products and individual differences in response account for the preferences we see in the clinical setting.

USE FOR Improving attention, antioxidant protection of DHA and phospholipids in brain cell membranes, improved microcirculation to the brain, reduction of histamine release and edema, better visual adaptation, protection of vitamin C.

HOW MUCH? *Grape Seed OPCs*
> Children: 50 mg per day
> Adults: 75 mg twice per day
> *Pine Bark OPCs*
> Children: 1 mg per pound of body weight, taken twice per day
> Adults: 1 mg per pound of body weight, taken twice per day

Vitamin C must be taken with OPCs in a ratio of ten parts Vitamin C to one part OPCs (Vitamin C 500 mg: 50 mg OPCs).

MINERALS

PRODUCT *Albion chelates of calcium, magnesium, copper, iron, zinc, selenium, chromium, and potassium*

Amino acid chelation is the process used by plants to sequester or capture minerals they absorb from the earth. Albion Laboratories in Clearfield, Utah, has focused on amino acid chelate research for forty years and has built extensive relationships with research facilities throughout the world. They are the most reliable source of amino-acid-chelated minerals and have done comprehensive absorption and bioavailability comparisons between Albion chelates and other mineral forms.

USE FOR To replace low levels of calcium, magnesium, zinc, iron, chromium, and potassium, and to enhance brain function.

HOW MUCH? *Calcium amino acid chelate*
> Children: 250 mg per day
> Adolescents: 750 mg per day
> Adults: 500 mg per day
> Pregnant and Lactating Women: 750 mg per day

> *Magnesium amino acid chelate*
> Children: 250 mg per day for 30 days, then down to 150 mg
> Adolescents: 500 mg per day for 30 days, then down to 300 mg

Adults: 500 mg per day for 30 days, then down to 300 mg
Pregnant and Lactating Women: 750 mg per day for 30
days, then down to 500 mg

Zinc amino acid chelate
Children: 10 mg per day for 30 days, then down to 5 mg daily
Adolescents: 15 mg per day for 30 days, then down to 10 mg
Pregnant and Lactating Women: 15 mg per day for 30 days,
then down to 10 mg

Iron amino acid chelate
Children: 10 mg per day
Adolescents and Adults: 15 mg per day
Pregnant and Lactating Women: 15 mg per day

Potassium amino acid chelate
Potassium is a necessary part of the *30-Day Plan*. After thirty
days, you can adjust the amount of potassium, depending on
your diet, ambient temperature, and amount of exercise you get.
If you use very little salt, are not perspiring much from exercise
or hot weather, or are retaining fluids, you may not need to continue potassium. Adults should not exceed 6 capsules per day and
no more than three taken at a single time. Children should take
no more than one at a time, and up to two per day.
Children: 2 capsules per day, one in the morning and the other
in the evening. Each capsule will contain 99 mg of potassium
Adolescents and Adults: 4 capsules per day, two in the
morning and two in the evening
Pregnant and Lactating Women: 4 capsules per day, two in
the morning and two in the evening

Copper amino acid chelate
Most homes today have copper pipes and you may already
have too much copper. You should have your hair tested for
copper levels before supplementing with this mineral.

Manganese amino acid chelate
Children: 1 capsule per day, 5 mg
Adults: 1 capsule per day, 15 mg

Chromium amino acid chelate
Chromium may be included in B-Stress formulas. If it is,
don't add extra.
Children: 100 mcg (micrograms) per day

Adolescents, Adults, Pregnant or Lactating Women: 200 mcg per day

Selenium (L-selenomethionine)
Selenium is usually included in antioxidant formulas. If so, don't add any extra.
Children: 50 mcg per day
Adolescents, Adults, Pregnant or Lactating Women: 200 mcg per day

B VITAMINS
PRODUCT *B Complex*

The B vitamins are essential cofactors for the enzymatic processes in the brain. You should take them together, and the supplement you choose should have extra B_6 or pyridoxine. Look for a capsule with these ratios:

B_1 *(thiamine HCl):* 25 mg
B_2 *(riboflavin):* 30 mg
B_3 *(niacinamide):* 50 mg
B_6 *(pyridoxine):* 50 mg
B_5 *(pantothenic acid):* 25 to 75 mg
B_{12} *(cobalamin):* 50 mcg
Folic acid: 200 mcg
Biotin: 50 to 75 mcg

You will probably also see choline and inositol in the vitamin B formula you choose. Stress formulas may have vitamin C, minerals, or herbs in them. If you select one of these formulas, make sure to count the minerals the formula contains into your daily totals. Always take B vitamins with food; otherwise they may upset your stomach.

HOW MUCH?

Children: 1 capsule daily with breakfast
Adolescents: 1 capsule with breakfast and one with dinner
Adolescents and Adults: 2 to 3 capsules daily depending on body size and need. Take with breakfast and dinner. Add a third capsule at lunch if you are taking three.

ANTIOXIDANTS
PRODUCT *Antioxidant formulas with vitamins A, C, E, and beta carotene*

You can select one of several good formulas from major supplement suppliers. Look for *natural* beta carotene, preferably in a full range of carotenoids including alpha carotene, lycopene, lutein, and zeaxanthin. A good multiple vitamin capsule will also supply these essential antioxidants and it will include vitamin D, which is not included in most antioxidant formulas. Look for the brands listed above under B vitamins that use Albion amino-acid-chelated minerals. You may only have to supplement with additional magnesium and potassium.

WHERE DO I GET THESE EXACT COMBINATIONS?

You will be able to get a good multiple vitamin and Albion chelated mineral formula that comes very close to my recommendations. The dosage for such a formula is about 6 capsules per day for adults and three a day for children. Add to this extra magnesium, vitamin C, Masquelier's OPC, Berkem's OPC Gold or Pycnogenol, fatty acids, and digestive enzymes. A nutrition specialist in the natural foods store you pick will be glad to help you get the brands I have listed above and work out the amounts for each member of your family.

Herbs, Amino Acids and Metabolites You will no doubt run across formulas that contain these items. I do no not include them in my *30-Day Plan* because the goal of *The ADD Nutrition Solution* is to correct AD/HD by reducing irritants and reversing nutrient deficits in brain cells.

However, herbs are extremely helpful for moderating the effects of AD/HD, and you may want to add them to your personal program. You can find excellent herbs to calm and promote sleep. I do not include them in my core program, however, because my focus is on alleviating the problem rather than addressing its symptoms. After the thirty-day period, herbs can be extremely useful in helping maintain normal stress levels, strengthen immunity, improve cognition and memory, and reduce the digestive distress and sleep problems associated with AD/HD.

Amino Acids, Melatonin, and 5-Hydroxytryptamine These substances are extremely targeted to specific imbalances in brain chemistry. If you do not know what the imbalances are, how can you address them? Better leave this determination to professionals. There are urinary tests that can easily determine what deficiencies or imbalances exist among these precursors and metabolites. Remember, not everyone with AD/HD has the same cluster of problems.

Melatonin and serotonin (5-HTP) are metabolites that the body produces. Melatonin regulates daily biorhythms and sleep/wake cycles. Serotonin is a calming neurotransmitter and low levels are associated with aggression and anxiety. High levels are often seen in autism. Amino acids including L-tyrosine, L-phenylalanine, L-glutamine, glycine, L-histidine, and DL methionine are precursors of neurotransmitters.

The *30-Day Plan* will balance out most of the problems common to individuals with AD/HD, and the supplements I recommend are extremely safe. If further accommodation for faulty neurotransmission needs to be made, your health-care provider should be the one to have these tests done and design an appropriate program.

Phosphatidyl choline is available as a supplement and AD/HD adults who are experiencing memory problems may find addition of this supplement very helpful. You may recall that phosphatidyl choline is the specific anchor for DHA in neurons.

An interesting paper on the use of two dietary supplements was published in the January/March 1998 edition of *Integrative Physiological and Behavioral Science*. Kathryn Dykman and Roscoe Dykman reported on a double-blind study in which they compared cognitive abilities among 17 AD/HD children who were given dietary supplements. The subjects were divided into three groups, those who were not on Ritalin, those whose Ritalin dose was cut in half, and those who were maintained on their usual Ritalin dose. All of the children were given a complex *glyconutritional* supplement for six weeks. A second phytonutritional supplement was added in the final three weeks of the trial. The research team reported an overall reduction in AD/HD symptom severity and associated oppositional and conduct disorders during the time the children were supplemented with the glyconutritional formula. There was no further improvement upon addition of the phytonutrient supplement.

I have had no first-hand experience with these dietary supplements, but I have had some clients who have reported a positive response to them. While these results look promising, the supplements in question might be *added* to my *30-Day Plan* to help overcome symptoms, but they do not contain the nutrients necessary to reverse the imbalances and deficiencies we have seen are at the root of AD/HD symptoms.

If you or your child is currently taking medication for AD/HD, do not discontinue its use. Work with your doctor to monitor the response to the medication. Abrupt withdrawal can have serious consequences. As the dietary change and nutrients begin to improve brain function, your doctor may adjust or discontinue the use of stimulants and other medications.

Some children have already been placed on Ritalin-free holidays—during weekends and summer vacation. If this is the case, it may be easier to discontinue the medication. Summertime is an ideal time to begin the *30-Day Plan* because there will be plenty of time for your child to get the full benefits of the plan before school begins again.

The AD/HD Diet: What to Eat and When to Eat It

Now that we have gone through all the foods and ingredients to avoid and what you *should* eat, how do you combine them and create a convenient daily dietary plan? I have designed a unique approach to better eating for your family and avoidance of harmful foods and ingredients that is easy to follow. I will provide a general plan and then make suggestions in regard to meal planning and shopping that will help you put it into action quickly and easily.

WHAT YOU SHOULD EAT DAILY TO REDUCE AD/HD EFFECTS

You should use the following guidelines to create a healthy combination of carbohydrates, proteins, and fats. I have outlined a plan here that regulates the balance of these three groups throughout the day with the most benefits to those with AD/HD.

- Carbohydrates: eat whole complex ones (grains, legumes, vegetables, fruit)

   No sugar or artificial sweeteners; limit fruit juice and natural sweeteners

   Balance with proteins 40% carbohydrates:30% proteins morning and midday; eat more in evening, 70% carbohydrates:20% proteins

- Proteins: eat high-quality proteins, fish, poultry, lamb, legumes, grains, vegetables, limit beef and pork, no eggs or dairy products during the *30-Day Plan*
    Balance 40:30 with carbohydrates morning and midday; Eat less in the evening, 70%carbohydrates: 20% protein
    Avoid potential allergens by consuming organic foods whenever possible, and use digestive enzymes to help avoid allergic reactions

- Fats:
    - Eliminate all hydrogenated and trans fats, dairy fats (except butter), and fried foods
    - Reduce saturated fats
    - Use olive, canola, nut oils, and Sunshine Butter as added fats
    - Choose tuna, salmon, herring, cod, menhaden, or trout, as much as possible; eat fish at least two times a week to get the fatty acids you need
    - Children should not be on low-fat or fat-free programs; adults should be on low-fat, but not on fat-free
    - Use added fats (oils, butter, nut butters) at two meals daily
- The Daily Menu Guides in chapter 15 provide for the following overall scheme:

- Breakfast: ⅓ daily carbohydrate servings, ⅔ protein, and 1 fat (morning snack)
- Lunch: ⅓ daily carbohydrate servings, ⅔ protein, fat optional (afternoon snack)
- Dinner ⅔ daily carbohydrate servings, ⅓ protein, fat optional (evening snack)

WHAT YOU SHOULD ELIMINATE FROM YOUR DIET

My *30-Day Plan* is designed to make implementing dietary changes simple. We will eliminate the foods and additives that science has revealed are most likely to cause problems. There can be as many as 500 additives in food at any one time, according to a national press survey. You or your child may be overwhelmed by the processed food you are eating. The cleaner you can get your diet, the fewer problems you will likely have. My shopping guide, menu plans, and substitution charts will show you how to easily work around these symptom-provoking substances. These are the items likely to affect your child's brain (more detail in appendix 1):

Foods: dairy products, dairy components (casein, lactalbumin, whey, lactose), chocolate, egg whites, wheat, corn, oranges, and peanuts

Sweeteners: sugar (cane or beet) and refined starches (corn syrup, corn starch, modified food starch, maltodextrin), high fructose corn syrup, all artificial sweeteners (NutraSweet, Equal, Sweet 'n Low, Sucralose, Acesulfame K)

Additives: try to eliminate all artificial colors, but especially red dye #3
   (erythrosine) and yellow dye #5 (tartrazine) which are the most studied and
   proven to exacerbate AD/HD
Flavors: MSG, vanillin, and smoke flavoring are the most common; avoid salt,
   sodium-containing agents, and sodium or potassium phosphate (buffering
   agents)
Preservatives: BHA, BHT, TBHQ, sodium benzoate, calcium propionate, nitrates
   and nitrites, sulfites, and citric acid
Beverages: all caffeinated tea, coffee, and sodas; sweetened fruit juices and
   beverages; and all others that contain phosphates
Fats: all hydrogenated and partially hydrogenated fats, mono and diglycerides,
   Olestra, Olean, tropical fats (palm, palm kernel, coconut), cottonseed oil

A CLOSER LOOK AT WHAT YOU SHOULD EAT FOR 30 DAYS

My *30-Day Plan* is nutritionally balanced to deliver 40 percent of the daily calories you eat as complex carbohydrates. These foods are listed under Starches and include cereals, bread, whole grains, many snack foods, legumes, and starchy vegetables. These foods contain five times the amount of carbohydrate to proteins and contain very little, albeit *good*, fat.

Green and leafy vegetables are listed under Veggies, although they also contain protein and carbohydrates, as do the starches. Here the carbohydrate to protein ratio is 2.5:1. Broccoli, cauliflower, celery, and sweet peppers all belong to this group.

Soy Milk Products as a group contribute carbohydrate, protein, and fats to the daily total. This group includes organic soy milk items, cheese, and yogurt.

The Fruits, Juices, Sweeteners category contains pure carbohydrates. Fruit, and especially fruit juices, can contribute a significant amount of carbohydrates, mostly sugars, to the daily quota. It is important to include fresh fruit in your diet because they contain valuable micronutrients, but I moderate their use to avoid aggravating AD/HD symptoms. Many children are drinking too much fruit juice and are getting too many sugars. Rice milk counts in this group, but it does contain protein and so can be consumed more often than fruit juice.

The remaining two food groups contain fats and proteins. Thirty percent of daily calories are designated for each of these categories in my plan. Thirty percent dietary fat content is considered a worthy health goal for Americans. Most of us eat a far higher percentage of fat calories daily. As you work with my menu plans, you will see how easy it is to add too many fats to your diet. Recommended fats are two-third oils and spreads and one-third Sunshine Butter. Avoid high-fat foods like bacon, sausage, and ham. You can eat these foods after you have been on my plan for thirty days, but only if you buy preservative-free and low-salt brands. You will also get some fats with the concentrated protein foods. Remember that children need more fat than do adults, but make sure they are eating the correct fats.

The protein levels I am recommending are high in comparison to traditional diet plans you may have seen, but eating good high-quality protein foods like fish, poultry, legumes, and soy foods, and ensuring their proper digestion, is a key element in overcoming AD/HD. The digestive system and brain are closely linked. Norepinephrine and acetylcholine, which are two of the most important neurotransmitters in the brain, are also active in digestion. Dozens of messages pass between the brain, sensory organs, and digestive system before, during, and after eating. Important clues about the nature of the food to be eaten, its chemical composition, and its digestive requirements are exchanged just by smelling or seeing the food! Once it enters your mouth, receptors on your tongue confirm its identity and further enhance the information needed for your body to digest the food.

FOR BEST RESULTS—SIT DOWN, RELAX, AND CHEW!

Our habit of eating on the run is a disaster for our digestive systems. Conflict during eating is another source of digestive problems. The conflict may come from unexpected sources, like the evening news, or reading the newspaper while eating. Most of us recognize that heated debate or arguing does not promote enjoyment of a meal and good digestion. It is important to remedy these situations for long-term success, and I urge you to examine how you eat meals in your home and make the necessary adjustments to make them as relaxing, calm, and pleasant as they can be.

When you are stressed, norepinephrine and epinephrine (adrenalin) shut down digestive processes because they are diverting energy to the brain and nervous system that would otherwise be expended digesting your meal. We have already seen how norepinephrine overcomes glucose deficits in the brain, and it will do the same in stressful situations. I can't imagine a worse scenario than sitting in traffic with your adrenalin running on high, while eating a hamburger and drinking coffee. Yet, millions of us do it daily. To digest the nutrients you need from the food you eat, this kind of behavior must stop.

When in doubt, use common sense. Think about what and when you are eating, and carefully follow my guidelines for thirty days. What should you do after thirty days? We'll discuss that later, but for now, here's the plan.

MENU PLANS

This is the basic menu plan for people of various ages. Choose the particular one that is appropriate for you. it shows you what food group should be eaten at a given time of day. There are six food groups. Serving sizes are also given in these lists. For example, the standard serving for a starchy food is one-half cup. I provide guidelines for the number of servings required for males and females, ages one through fifty, in chapter 12. Next, refer to the substitution food lists and select the foods you can rotate into the sample plan for variety. You should try to follow these recommendations and schedule eating times as close to the same time as you can each day.

SERVING SIZES

STARCHES	FRUIT	VEGGIES	SOY MILK PRODUCTS	PROTEINS	FAT
Serving size = ½ cup	Serving size = ½ medium fruit. Fruit Juice serving size= ½ cup. Sweeteners serving size = 1 teaspoon.	Serving size = ½ cup cooked or juiced or 1 cup raw	Serving size = 1 cup	Serving size = 1 ounce	Serving Size = 1 teaspoon

DAILY SERVINGS FOR CHILDREN 1 TO 3 YEARS

MEALS	STARCHES 1 = ½ cup	FRUIT 1 = ½ medium JUICE 1 = ½ cup SWEETENERS 1 = 1 tsp	VEGGIES 1 = ½ cup cooked or 1 cup raw	SOY MILK PRODUCTS 1 = 1 cup	PROTEINS 1 = 1 oz	FATS 1 = one tsp
Breakfast	½	1		½	2	
Mid-Morning Snack			½			

MEALS	STARCHES 1 = ½ cup	FRUIT 1 = ½ medium JUICE 1 = ½ cup SWEETENERS 1 = 1 tsp	VEGGIES 1 = ½ cup cooked or 1 cup raw	SOY MILK PRODUCTS 1 = 1 cup	PROTEINS 1 = 1 oz	FATS 1 = one tsp
Lunch	½		1	½	2	1
After-School Snack	1		½		1	
Dinner	2		1	1	3	2
Bedtime Snack		1				
Totals	4	2	3	2	8	3

DAILY SERVINGS FOR CHILDREN 4 TO 6 YEARS

MEALS	STARCHES 1 = ½ cup	FRUIT 1 = ½ medium JUICE 1 = ½ cup SWEETENERS 1 = 1 tsp	VEGGIES 1 = ½ cup cooked or 1 cup raw	SOY MILK PRODUCTS 1 = 1 cup	PROTEINS 1 = 1 oz	FATS 1 = one tsp
Breakfast	1	1		1	3	
Mid-Morning Snack			1			
Lunch	1		1	1	3	2
After-School Snack	1		1		3	
Dinner	3		1	1	3	3
Bedtime Snack		2				
Totals	6	3	4	3	12	5

DAILY SERVINGS FOR CHILDREN 7 TO 10 YEARS

MEALS	STARCHES 1 = ½ cup	FRUIT 1 = ½ medium JUICE 1 = ½ cup SWEETENERS 1 = 1 tsp	VEGGIES 1 = ½ cup cooked or 1 cup raw	SOY MILK PRODUCTS 1 = 1 cup	PROTEINS 1 = 1 oz	FATS 1 = one tsp
Breakfast	1	2		1	4	
Mid-Morning Snack			1			

DAILY SERVINGS FOR CHILDREN 7 TO 10 YEARS (continued)

MEALS	STARCHES 1 = ½ cup	FRUIT 1 = ½ medium JUICE 1 = ½ cup SWEETENERS 1 = 1 tsp	VEGGIES 1 = ½ cup cooked or 1 cup raw	SOY MILK PRODUCTS 1 = 1 cup	PROTEINS 1 = 1 oz	FATS 1 = one tsp
Lunch	1		1	1	3	2
After-School Snack	1		1		4	
Dinner	4		2	2	3	3
Bedtime Snack		2				
Totals	7	4	5	4	14	5

DAILY SERVINGS FOR BOYS 11 TO 14 YEARS

MEALS	STARCHES 1 = ½ cup	FRUIT 1 = ½ medium JUICE 1 = ½ cup SWEETENERS 1 = 1 tsp	VEGGIES 1 = ½ cup cooked or 1 cup raw	SOY MILK PRODUCTS 1 = 1 cup	PROTEINS 1 = 1 oz	FATS 1 = one tsp
Breakfast	2	2		2	5	1
Mid-Morning Snack			1			
Lunch	2		2	1	3	2
After-School Snack			1		3	
Dinner	4		2	2	5	3
Bedtime Snack		3				
Totals	8	5	6	5	16	6

DAILY SERVINGS FOR GIRLS 11 TO 18 YEARS AND ADULT WOMEN UP TO AGE 50

MEALS	STARCHES 1 = ½ cup	FRUIT 1 = ½ medium JUICE 1 = ½ cup SWEETENERS 1 = 1 tsp	VEGGIES 1 = ½ cup cooked or 1 cup raw	SOY MILK PRODUCTS 1 = 1 cup	PROTEINS 1 = 1 oz	FATS 1 = one tsp
Breakfast	1	2		1	4	
Mid-Morning Snack			1			
Lunch	1		2	1	4	2
After-School Snack	1		1		4	
Dinner	4		2	2	3	3
Bedtime Snack		2				
Totals	7	4	6	4	15	5

DAILY SERVINGS FOR MALES 15 TO 18 YEARS

MEALS	STARCHES 1 = ½ cup	FRUIT 1 = ½ medium JUICE 1 = ½ cup SWEETENERS 1 = 1 tsp	VEGGIES 1 = ½ cup cooked or 1 cup raw	SOY MILK PRODUCTS 1 = 1 cup	PROTEINS 1 = 1 oz	FATS 1 = one tsp
Breakfast	3	2		2	6	1
Mid-Morning Snack			1			
Lunch	3		2	2	3	2
After-School Snack	1	2	1		3	
Dinner	5		3	2	6	3
Bedtime Snack		2				
Totals	12	6	7	6	18	6

DAILY SERVINGS FOR MALES 19+ YEARS

MEALS	STARCHES 1 = ½ cup	FRUIT 1 = ½ medium JUICE 1 = ½ cup SWEETENERS 1 = 1 tsp	VEGGIES 1 = ½ cup cooked or 1 cup raw	SOY MILK PRODUCTS 1 = 1 cup	PROTEINS 1 = 1 oz	FATS 1 = one tsp
Breakfast	3	3		2	5	2
Mid-Morning Snack			1			
Lunch	2		2	1	5	2
Afternoon Snack	1		1			
Dinner	7		4	1	6	3
Bedtime Snack		3				
Totals	13	6	8	4	16	7

DAILY SERVINGS FOR PREGNANT WOMEN IN THE 2ND AND 3RD TRIMESTER

MEALS	STARCHES 1 = ½ cup	FRUIT 1 = ½ medium JUICE 1 = ½ cup SWEETENERS 1 = 1 tsp	VEGGIES 1 = ½ cup cooked or 1 cup raw	SOY MILK PRODUCTS 1 = 1 cup	PROTEINS 1 = 1 oz	FATS 1 = one tsp
Breakfast	2	2		2	3	
Mid-Morning Snack			1			1
Lunch	1	1	2	1	4	2
Afternoon Snack	1		1		3	
Dinner	4		2	2	6	3
Bedtime Snack		2				
Totals	8	5	6	5	16	6

DAILY SERVINGS FOR NURSING MOTHERS

MEALS	STARCHES I = ½ cup	FRUIT I = ½ medium JUICE I = ½ cup SWEETENERS I = I tsp	VEGGIES I = ½ cup cooked or I cup raw	SOY MILK PRODUCTS I = I cup	PROTEINS I = I oz	FATS I = one tsp
Breakfast	2	2		2	4	2
Mid-Morning Snack			I			
Lunch	2	2	2	I	4	2
Afternoon Snack	I		I			
Dinner	4		4	2	8	3
Bedtime Snack		2				
Totals	9	6	8	5	16	7

Now, how do you fill in your grid with actual foods? Here is one of the menu plans with the kind of food and size of serving I suggest. The sample plan charts daily servings in each food group required by children seven to ten years of age. You can compare it to the menu plan for children of other ages and for your own menu plan. Note each box in the grid tallies the number of food servings included in the box. In some cases, servings from more than one food group are listed because they are included in food preparation. For example, confetti rice includes equal portions of uncooked rice and mixed vegetables. The menu plan also gives an accounting of what food group it's from and how much you can subtract from the daily total when you eat it. I share the recipes for the foods included in the grid in chapter 17. Complete lists of substitution foods are given in chapter 17.

The first menu plan works around the main meal of the day; in this case it is the Traditional Meat, Starch, and Veggie Plan.

SAMPLE DAILY MENU PLAN—TRADITIONAL MEAT, STARCH, AND VEGGIE (MSV)

NOTE: SERVING SIZES ARE FOR CHILDREN 7 TO 10 YEARS.

MEALS	STARCHES	FRUIT	VEGGIES	SOY MILK PRODUCTS	PROTEINS	FATS
Breakfast	½ cup oatmeal (=1 starch)	½ cup fresh strawberries, halved (=1 fruit)		½ cup flavored soy milk (=½ soy)	Smoothie with ½ cup soy yogurt and ½ cup pineapple juice (= 4 Protein, 1 fruit, ½ soy)	
Mid-Morning Snack			packet of baby carrots (=1 veggie)			
Lunch	one slice oatmeal bread (=1 starch)		3 cherry tomatoes (=1 veggie)	1 boxed soy beverage (=1 soy)	3 ounces lean turkey breast (=3 protein)	½ Tbsp mayonnaise (=½ fat)
After-School Snack	1 slice rice bread with tuna salad mixture (=1 starch)		4 small broccoli trees with miso dip (=1 veggie, ½ fat)		Two rounded tablespoons tuna salad (=4 protein, 1 fat)	
Dinner	1 cup steamed confetti rice, ½ cup cooked acorn squash (=4 starch, 1 veggie)		½ cup steamed spinach with nutmeg (=1 veggie, 1 fat)	2 cups of soy milk (=2 soy)	3 oz baked fillet of sole (=3 protein)	2 tsp of olive oil used in preparation of dishes (=2 fat)
Bedtime Snack		1 medium banana (=2 fruit)				
Totals	7	4	5	4	14	5

Now, what do you do if you are planning a main dish for dinner? This plan, which I call the One-Dish Meal, or ODM, is based on a dinner casserole, Italian Beef and Vegetables. You will find the recipe in chapter 16. It is very easy to slip a favorite casserole into the daily menu plan. There are many variations for this dish and it is one of the mainstays of family dining. As long as the proportions of pasta, vegetables, oil, cheese, and beef are kept constant, you can vary the presentation many ways. Experiment with different seasonings and types of pasta to lend different flavors.

SAMPLE DAILY MENU PLAN—ONE-DISH MEAL (ODM)

Note: Serving Sizes are for Children 7 to 10 years						
MEALS	STARCHES	FRUIT	VEGGIES	SOY MILK PRODUCTS	PROTEINS	FATS
Breakfast	½ cup mutli-grain cereal (wheat-free, corn-free) (=1 starch)	½ cup fresh strawberries, halved (=1 fruit)		½ cup flavored soy milk (=½ soy, other ½) in smoothie	Smoothie with ½ cup soy yogurt and ½ cup pineapple juice (= 4 protein, 1 fruit, ½ soy)	
Mid-Morning Snack			packet of baby carrots (=1 veggie)			
Lunch	1 slice oatmeal bread (=1 starch)		5 cherry tomatoes (= 1¾ veggie)	1 boxed soy beverage (=1 soy)	3 ounces lean turkey breast (=3 protein)	2 tsp mustard
After school Snack	1 slice rice bread (=1 starch)		4 small broccoli trees (=1 veggie)		Two tablespoons tuna salad (=3 protein, 1 fat)	(1 fat in tuna salad)
Dinner	1 starch in casserole + 1½ cups green peas=3 starch		1¼ in casserole	1 cup soy milk (=1 soy)	4 proteins in casserole	4 fat in casserole
Bedtime Snack		1 medium banana +1 tbsp honey 1 starch (=2 fruit)		1 cup soy yogurt		
Totals	7	4	5	4	14	5

Macaroni and cheese tops most children's list of favorite meals. I will now show you how easy it is to adapt the ODM plan for a starchy meal like macaroni and cheese with my recipe as a substitute for kids' usual boxed variety favorite. Spaghetti and meatballs, pizza, or hearty cream soups fit just as easily into this plan. The oatmeal cookie in this plan can be an oatmeal cookie you bake with my guidelines in mind or any from the pantry management suggestions in the appendices. This same menu plan can be used for another family favorite, creamed tuna and baked potatoes. Again, recipes for these dishes can be found in chapter 17.

SAMPLE DAILY MENU PLAN—STARCHY ONE-DISH MEAL (SODM)

Note: Serving Sizes are for Children 7 to 10 years						
MEALS	STARCHES	FRUIT	VEGGIES	SOY MILK PRODUCTS	PROTEINS	FATS
Breakfast	½ cup granola (sugar-free, oil-free) (= 1 starch)	½ cup fresh strawberries, halved (= 1 fruit)		½ cup flavored soy milk (= ½ soy, other ½ in smoothie)	Smoothie with ½ cup soy yogurt and ½ cup pineapple juice (= 4 protein, 1 fruit, ½ soy)	
Mid-Morning Snack			packet of mixed veggies (= 1 veggie)			
Lunch	one slice oatmeal bread (= 1 starch)		5 cherry tomatoes (= 1¾ veggie)	1 boxed soy beverage (=1 soy)	3 ounces lean turkey breast (= 3 protein)	1 tsp mayo (= 1 fat)
After-School Snack	1 slice rice bread (= 1 starch)		4 small broccoli trees, with miso dip (= 1 veggie)		Four tablespoons tuna salad (= 5 protein, 1 fat)	1 fat in tuna salad, 1 fat in dip (= 2 fat)
Dinner	1 cup macaroni 2 starch in casserole		1½ cups mixed veggies in salad	2 cups soy milk (= 2 soy)	2 proteins in cheese and soy milk	2 fats in cheese
Bedtime Snack	1 oatmeal cookie (= 2 starch)	1 cup fruit juice or rice milk (= 2 fruit)				
Totals	7	4	5	4	14	5

Children can easily learn how to work with the basic menu plan, and it is a great tool for teaching them how to eat a healthy diet. We are building a drug-free future for our AD/HD children—and ourselves!

Toward this end, I suggest you remove the appropriate basic menu plan for yourself or your child and slip it inside a plastic page protector. Post it someplace convenient and keep a washable marker nearby. Plan in the evening what you will eat the next day or days and then cross off the appropriate box as each food is eaten. You will become proficient at tallying what you have eaten and what you have left to eat. Children become expert at this, but watch out because they also become experts at negotiating their way around what they should eat!

Now that you are comfortable with using the menu plans for designing your meals, a simple food substitution list is given below.

MENU PLAN FOOD SUBSTITUTIONS

STARCHES	FRUIT	VEGGIES	SOY MILK PRODUCTS	PROTEINS	FAT
Serving size = ½ cup	Serving size = ½ medium fruit. Fruit Juice serving size= ½ cup. Sweeteners serving size = 1 teaspoon.	Serving size = ½ cup cooked or juiced or 1 cup raw	Serving size = 1 cup soy or rice	Serving size = 1 ounce	Serving Size = 1 teaspoon
hot and cold cereals (not sweetened), rice, pasta, potatoes, corn, peas, yams, winter squash, lentils, beans Crackers 2 medium Rice Cakes 1 large Tortilla 1 medium Muffins 1 small	apples, pears, cherries, figs, berries, mangoes, pineapples, kiwis, bananas, etc.	All green and yellow veggies, except those listed under starches, tomato sauce and tomato juice Carrot juice, ½ cup Salad greens 2 cups raw	soy milk, soy yogurt, soy sour cream	lean beef, pork, lamb, poultry, fish, shellfish **Vegetarian Choices** Tofu, Tempeh 4 oz or 1 slice 2½" x 2¾" x 1" Legumes, cooked, ½ cup Hummus 4 tablespoons	butter, oils, 1 slice bacon Salad Dressing (creamy type) 1 Tbs Nuts ¼ cup Nut Butters 1 Tbs Cheese-High Fat 1 oz

MENU FOOD PLAN SUBSTITUTIONS *(continued)*

STARCHES	FRUIT	VEGGIES	SOY MILK PRODUCTS	PROTEINS	FAT
Serving size = ½ cup	Serving size = ½ medium fruit. Fruit Juice serving size= ½ cup. Sweeteners serving size = 1 teaspoon.	Serving size = ½ cup cooked or juiced or 1 cup raw	Serving size = 1 cup	Serving size = 1 ounce	Serving Size = 1 teaspoon
Pancakes 2 four-inch					

Condiments (count as carbohydrates) serving size = ¼ cup barbecue sauce, ketchup; 1½ Tbs tartar sauce; 2 Tbs miso

Now that we have the menu plans explained and you have the tools to begin my *30-Day Plan*, you are probably wondering what to do *after* the thirty days. And what about eating out or choosing prepared foods?

EATING OUT AND TAKE-OUT MEALS

One of the fastest growing trends in the United States is "home-meal replacement," which is a new name for meals prepared outside your own kitchen. In 1996, Americans forked over more than three billion dollars for meals prepared for them outside their homes. This represents an amazing 46 percent of the total dollars spent on food. Meals purchased outside the home were equally divided between take-out food and restaurant dining.

In many homes today, both parents work and children are car-pooled to after-school activities such as soccer, swimming, and gymnastics. It leaves little time for food preparation, prompting some families to rely on home-meal replacements for up to half the family meals.

Supermarket delis are a growing phenomenon, convenient and profitable. I discuss the nutritional hazards lurking within these departments, and how to avoid them, in chapter 16. Supermarkets are touting their menus and specials on the Internet in an effort to win food dollars away from fast-growing chains of prepared food service. Gelson's, an upscale market in southern California, carries entrees from restaurant chef Wolfgang Puck. And Ukrop's chain, based in Richmond, Virginia, has devoted 45 percent of the floor space in its stores to prepared foods. Natural food chains, like Wild Oats, Whole Foods, and Fresh Fields, have catered to the gourmet tastes of health-conscious consumers with prepared meals, many of them vegetarian, since the mid-1980s.

It all started with Boston Market's rotisserie chicken back in the early 1980s. More "personalized meals" are also available, with entire menus prepared "just like Mom would fix." Still confined to smaller companies, this type of service offers whole meals, including main dish, salad, dessert and beverage, with home delivery—even at a distance.

There is a big difference in the quality of food you get from these various establishments. Some are "safe" for AD/HD individuals, others are not. A recent shopping trip to our local supermarket chain revealed a list of ingredients that barely fit onto the label of a "Healthy Choice" side dish in their deli. The service deli counter did not have an ingredient list for any of the items they were serving up, nor did they understand why I needed this information.

We decided to try a smaller shop in our neighborhood that specializes in cooked foods to take home and heat. Perhaps a smaller, friendlier business and one that is catering to a family community would be more helpful. The entrees were not that tasty, despite rave reviews in the local paper, and the head clerk was not any more forthcoming with ingredient lists than the supermarket. If I wanted to know, I was informed, I would have to present a list of what to avoid and they would go into the back room and check their recipes. Can you imagine how inconvenient that would be at dinnertime when the shop fills with customers?

We had a more pleasant experience, on the other hand, when we ordered an organic dinner recently from Diamond Organics in Freedom, California. We were delighted with the quality, flavor, and price of the meal. The organic baby greens were the freshest we've seen and the serving sizes were just right. We declined the bottle of wine they offered, but for the ultimate dining experience—why not? Most importantly, Diamond readily discloses their ingredient list so you can avoid allergy trigger foods. They deliver anywhere in the United States, but you have to plan a day ahead for next-day FedEx delivery.

Now what about eating out? You should apply the same diligence in selecting foods in a restaurant as you do at home. I have found that most good restaurants will gladly modify existing menu selections to meet your specifications. A pretty safe bet is to ask for a vegetarian plate. Just make sure they don't add sauces or seasoning other than herbs. If you have determined that you or your child is sensitive to many cooking spices or condiments, take your own seasoning along to add to your meal at the restaurant. Avoid fast-food restaurants because the food is often mass-produced with unknown additives and the servers usually cannot help you identify them. A small local family-owned restaurant is often a great choice for a family with young children.

AFTER THE THIRTY DAYS

You have no doubt noticed great improvement in the way you feel or in your child's behavior as you approach your thirtieth day on the plan. You may have noticed less fatigue, improved skin condition, absence of dark circles and swelling around the eyes, in addition to improved behavior and attention. The dietary changes you have made removed most of the trigger foods that were causing these symptoms.

Now, how do you determine which ones these are so you can broaden your food choices as much as possible? Once your body has not confronted a trigger food for thirty days, it will react when that food is reintroduced into the diet. There are several ways you can proceed to identify problem foods. Physicians who specialize in food sensitivities can be located by calling one of the medical associations listed in the appendix. You will need to find a doctor who uses provocation techniques, RAST, FICA, or ELISA testing. Once the trigger foods are identified, sublingual drops can be prepared to desensitize your child, so that the trigger foods can be eaten without causing a problem.

Another way to work around trigger foods is to identify them with the help of a doctor and then rotate the offending food so that it is not eaten more frequently than every four days.

The last method is to do it yourself, although I do not recommend this. The eliminated foods are tested—one at a time—by introducing a new one every four days and observing the child for a reaction. Typical reactions are flushing, rapid pulse, change in behavior, mood swings, and anxiety. These can be difficult to detect, which is why I recommend you work with a professional. You have spent a lot of time and effort on the *30-Day Plan* and have reduced symptoms by eliminating offending foods and additives. Your child will be very sensitive to testing or reintroduction of these foods at this time. Therefore, it is the best time to identify trigger foods. More detail on the home-detection method is given below.

As for additives, you will want to eliminate them entirely from your diet for the long term. You will have to observe both your own and your child's response to occasional encounters with additives. My experience is that most children and some adults will continue to have neurological symptoms with additives. Children soon learn this, and after a symptom-free month, your child will not like the way he or she feels after eating too many sugars, colorings, or flavors. As an adult you will most likely be much more selective about what you eat, once you've identified foods or additives that make you feel tense, anxious, sluggish, forgetful, depressed, or short-tempered.

CHALLENGING WITH FOOD ELIMINATED DURING THE 30-DAY PLAN

The *30-Day Plan* is modeled after the clinical trials I described in previous chapters and you have just completed the *elimination phase* with the *30-Day Plan*. Your or your child's symptoms will have improved immensely and you will understand how important diet and supplements are in beating AD/HD.

We are now ready to begin to *challenge* the body by reintroducing some of the foods you have eliminated during the thirty days, to identify which are causing the problem. We will test each of the foods, one at a time, every four days. This is the *challenge* phase. It is best to be working with a physician at this point, because identifying allergic response is extremely difficult. A new test for food immune complexes is available, which I described in chapter 9. A list of physician resources for food allergy testing can be found in appendix 4.

You will be looking for symptoms that the food just eaten is a problem. Serve a good-sized portion of the food to be tested without anything else except water. Here are the symptoms to watch for.

Symptoms
Immediate:
    runny nose shortly after eating the food
    itchy eyes
    sneezing or stuffy nose
    rapid pulse
    marked change in behavior
    increased anxiety
    red ears or cheeks
    change of mood, either elevated or depressed

Delayed Reaction:
    stomachache
    gas and bloating
    constipation and diarrhea
    dark circles under the eyes

    red eyes
    rash
    headache or muscle ache
    stuffy nose
    congestion
    listlessness
    change in behavior or mood

Carefully note any changes you observe, the time of day they occurred, how long after eating the food, and what food was eaten. If you note a response during the four-day period following the challenge, identify the provoking food as a trigger.

Four days later, repeat the process with another food and record the results. The entire challenge period will take a month. Continue with the same amounts of dietary supplements during the month. Follow this order of reintroduction:

    peanuts
    oranges
    sugar
    chocolate
    eggs
    corn
    wheat
    goat cheese, then cow's milk cheese, four days apart
    goat's or sheep's milk, then cow's milk, four days apart
    goat and cow's yogurt, buttermilk
    whole milk

In addition to these foods, adults will most likely want to test for their reaction to white wine, followed by red wine, if these items are consumed at all. If you have a corn allergy, whiskey made from corn can provoke symptoms, and it usually contains wheat as well. You may find you tolerate distilled spirits better than those that are not, but no alcoholic beverage can be tolerated by those with AD/HD except on an occasional basis.

THE LONG-TERM PLAN

After sixty days, you will have pretty well identified what your long-term nutrition program will include or avoid. Avoid trigger foods, rotate those on the list, continue to follow the menu plans, and avoid additives. You will be able to try eating out now and again, but question the restaurant carefully about use of preservatives, MSG, and other additives. You will want to eliminate eating trigger foods, even as ingredients. I know this takes time and effort, but your child's health, as well as your own, is at stake.

Take it very slowly and be patient. You will find that you or your child is getting stabilized and you can permit occasional transgressions. If your child does have a bad reaction after going to a birthday party or some other event, return to the strict *30-Day Plan* for four days.

After three months, you can begin to reduce the dietary supplements you or your child is on. Start by removing them on weekends, so you have a five-day-on two-day-off plan. Then one weekday decrease the fatty acids by half. Continue on the minerals, vitamins, and OPC or Pycnogenol. After two weeks, decrease a fatty acid capsule a second day. Keep reducing this supplement until you or your child is taking one fatty acid capsule per day, and a multivitamin mineral capsule five days out of seven. Each individual will respond a little differently and have different nutrient needs. You will be the best judge of what amounts of dietary supplements you or your child needs to feel and perform your best, based on your reaction to these reductions.

Once you discover what an impact diet has had on your AD/HD, you will probably never be able to eat the way you did before. Most people find it just isn't worth it.

Let's move on to shopping and what to choose for your shopping cart.

Your Personal Shopping Guide to Healthy Pantry Management

The first thing you will have to do to implement the *30-Day Plan* is to go through your cupboards and refrigerator and replace with alternatives those staples, snacks, condiments, and other items that we are trying to eliminate in this plan. The process will be considerably simplified because a complete list of what to avoid and why you should avoid them is included in chapter 17.

You will also find complete lists of brands to shop for in each food category and what kind of store is likely to have the specified item. Here's the overall plan in ten steps:

Ten steps you should follow to make the *30-Day Plan* work:

1. Clean and restock your pantry
2. Study the list in the appendices for what to avoid
3. Make up your shopping list and take it to the store with this book for reference
4. Select the stores you will shop in
5. Study the sample menus for when to eat proteins, carbohydrates, and fats

> 6. Check the recipe section, which will tell you how to make substitutions for favorite family recipes
> 7. Check the list of dietary supplements you will need to purchase
> 8. Refer to the mail-order list for hard-to-find items
> 9. Use the lists of professional associations for help in finding a nutritionally minded doctor in your area
> 10. Check out the references for support groups

PICK YOUR PLACE TO SHOP

You have no doubt discovered there is a big difference in supermarkets. Most of us look for convenience first and therefore check out the store closest to home. Convenience is important when you want to pick up a few last-minute items, but the closest market may not provide what you need to overcome AD/HD.

You are about to embark on a new shopping experience, and you will want to pick the most pleasant shopping environment so that you can take some time to scrutinize labels. You will have to find two kinds of stores to supply what you will need for the *30-Day Plan* and beyond.

The first is a good supermarket to supply most of your grocery needs. The second is a natural-foods store where you will find staples, supplements, and items that are hard to find at the grocery store. Depending on the size of your community, you may have a smaller health-food store that will carry the supplements you will need, but you may have to order staples. Mail-order businesses are listed in appendix 2 for you to use in this case. However, the demand for organic and specialty foods has been increasing so much that most communities have at least one large natural-foods market where you can do your entire shopping. Here are some tips about choosing quality stores to shop.

SHOP THE PERIMETER

Watching out for food additives is a challenge in today's modern supermarket. I often tell audiences, "Shop the perimeter of the store and stay out of the middle!" The reason for this shopping method is to avoid additives, preservatives, sugar, and fat. Nutrient-dense foods are located in the produce, dairy, and meat sections, which, in most supermarkets, are located around the perimeter. The only middle aisles you should visit are those that contain rice, paper goods, laundry and bath products, and frozen fruits and vegetables. You will have to be very selective in the cereal section. Most cereals contain sugar, wheat or corn, and additives that you are trying to avoid.

You will have to watch out for the bakeries and delis that are being added to the perimeter of larger stores. With few exceptions, items located there can only be purchased once in a while, not on a regular basis. Did you ever wonder why our stores are getting so much larger? What do they fill them with?

Supermarket managment has found bigger stores can accommodate huge profit centers that contain ready-to-eat and easily prepared gourmet and specialty foods. There is a great demand for these items from consumers who like the convenience and the status appeal of much of the imported goods in these aisles. However, high-end packaging or foreign production doesn't necessarily mean healthy, although food from other countries usually does have fewer additives than many of our U.S. brands. So, just remember to read the labels before you drop these items into your cart.

You pay a high price for the convenience of having food ready-to-go. Nevertheless, the convenience is well worth it sometimes—if you can navigate your way through the ingredients. The information in appendices 1 and 2 will guide you.

SUPPLEMENTS

The dietary supplements you will need for my *30-Day Plan* will be in your health or natural-foods store. These include fatty acids, vitamins, amino-acid-chelated minerals, and OPCs. It is important to the success of your program that you accept no substitutes for the specific products I recommend. I have been using and formulating dietary supplements for over thirty years. I have designed the supplement program to include only those items that are supported by research on their effectiveness in AD/HD and related disorders.

MAIL ORDER

Several companies offer direct mail for staples, produce, and supplements. If you like to stock up by mail, or if you do not have a natural foods or health-food store nearby, this can be very convenient. You will find the ordering information of companies that offer the most complete line of products listed in appendix 2.

What's in a Food Label?

Reading food labels can be intimidating. There are hundreds of differ-ent names for sugars, fats, and additives, and complete lists are located in appendix 1. I will go over several labels here that are representative of what you will find in most stores, and tell you what the ingredient is, its purpose, and whether it is approved for my *30-Day Plan*.

Put on Your Glasses and Read Those Labels!

Labeling of foods has gotten much more informative, thanks to the FDA revisions that were implemented between 1992 and 1993. You can now get information on the protein, carbohydrate, and fat content of a product, plus details on amounts of saturated, monounsaturated, and polyunsaturated fats each one contains. The fat breakdown is not required, but many labels do contain this valuable information. You may have paid little attention to this information—except possibly for the total fat grams—until now. An important part of my *30-Day Plan* is reading labels carefully. You will not want to put anything in your shop-ping cart that can be a trigger for your child's (or your own) AD/HD symptoms.

To help you do this, here is a representation of a cereal label and what it means—both the good and the bad!

Nutrition Facts

Serving Size ¾ cup (30 g)

Servings Per Container About 1.5

Amount Per Serving

Calories

 Calories from fat

	% Daily Value*
Total Fat 1.5 g†	2%
Saturated Fat 0 g	0%
Polyunsaturated Fat 0 g	
Monounsaturated Fat 0.5 g	
Cholesterol 0 mg	0%
Sodium 230 mg	10%
Total Carbohydrate 26 g	9%
Dietary Fiber 1 g	4%
Sugars 11 g	

	% Daily Value*
Protein 1 g	
Vitamin A	15%
Vitamin C	25%
Calcium	0%
Iron	25%
Vitamin D	0%
Thiamin	25%
Riboflavin	25%
Niacin	25%
Vitamin B$_6$	25%
Folic Acid	25%
Zinc	25%

*Percent Daily Values are based on a 2,000 calorie diet. Your daily value may be higher or lower depending on your calorie needs.

†Amount in cereal. One serving of cereal plus skim milk provides 1.5 g fat, less than 5 mg cholesterol, 300 mg sodium, 250 mg potassium, 32 g carbohydrates (17 g sugars), and 5 g protein.

FATS

The Nutrition Facts panel reveals that the cereal provides 2 percent of the fat requirement for 2,000 total daily calories. Ten percent of the total calories contained in the product come from fat. This isn't too bad and the fats are monounsaturated, which is good. Maddeningly, the government doesn't require trans-fat content to be listed in the Nutrition Facts panel. But you can determine the product's trans-fat content when the label lists monounsaturated and polyunsaturated fats in addition to saturated fat content. Simply add the amounts of these three fats and then subtract their sum from the total grams of fat. For this product, the total for the three fats is 0.5g. Subtracting this from the total fat grams listed (1.5g) gives a difference of 1 gram, which is the amount of trans fats. All labels are based on 2,000 calories and therefore provide good information for children ages seven to ten. Girls and women up to age fifty require 2,200 calories per day, and pregnant and lactating women require an additional 300 and 500 calories, respectively, per day. Males fifteen to eighteen will need 3,000 calories per day, and those nineteen to fifty need 2,800 calories.

CHOLESTEROL

There is no cholesterol in the cereal and adding soy milk, which is cholesterol free, wouldn't change this. However, if you added skim milk as suggested by the manufacturer, you would add the cholesterol contained in the milk. You may also recall that in chapter 12 I advised that children—even those without AD/HD—should not be offered *skim* milk. They need their brain fats, and of course those with AD/HD on my *30-Day Plan* should not have dairy at all.

CARBOHYDRATES AND SUGARS

The cereal provides over 10 percent of the daily carbohydrate requirements and almost half are sugars. Note that although the label reads 9 percent, carbohydrate calories in the *30-Day Plan* (40 percent) are less than what is allowed in a standard diet. The sugars in this product are especially harmful for those with AD/HD because they come from corn (corn syrup). This product contains some fiber, but it is from whole wheat, another no-no for the *30-Day Plan*.

SODIUM

Sodium content is 10 percent of the daily allowance, and it comes from salt, baking soda, vitamin C (sodium ascorbate), and trisodium phosphate (TSP). The TSP, an emulsifying and acidifying agent, is especially bad because it adds sodium *and* phosphate, both of which can interfere with mineral balance in the brain. (See chapter 11 for more discussion on phosphates.) TSP is often used for washing walls and woodwork, especially before painting, but it isn't especially desirable in food! Soy lecithin is a better and more natural emulsifying agent. Calcium and magnesium ascorbate are better forms of nonacidic vitamin C.

OVERALL INGREDIENTS

Now let's check the list of ingredients. It contains corn meal, whole wheat, modified corn starch, partially hydrogenated soybean oil, corn syrup, brown sugar syrup, salt, nonfat milk, baking soda, dextrose, cinnamon, trisodium phosphate, vitamin C (sodium ascorbate), zinc and iron, vitamin A (palmitate), and the B vitamins thiamine mononitrate (B_1), riboflavin (B_2), niacin, pyridoxine hydrochloride (B_6), and folic acid. Listed after niacin is blue 1 lake, and BHT is added for freshness.

Here's the breakdown:

THE GOOD	WHAT'S GOOD	THE BAD	WHAT'S BAD
Vitamin A Palmitate, B Vitamins, Vitamin C, Iron, and Zinc	Essential vitamins and minerals		Amounts of B vitamins are low and several important ones are missing. Most essential minerals are missing; must be provided elsewhere.
		Corn (meal, modified corn starch, corn syrup, dextrose)	Not included in *30-Day Plan*
		Wheat (graham)	Not included in *30-Day Plan*
		Nonfat milk	Not included in *30-Day Plan*
		Sugar (corn syrup, starch, brown sugar syrup, dextrose) is the second ingredient	Impacts brain function. Corn products not included in *30-Day Plan*
		Partially hydrogenated soybean oil and trans fats	Hydrogenated and trans fats block necessary brain fats.
		Sodium (salt, baking soda, trisodium phosphate, ascorbate)	Reduce availability of potassium, needed for brain and nerve transmission
		Artificial colors (blue lake 1) or preservatives (BHT)	Often worsen AD/HD symptoms
"contains wheat and milk products"	It is clearly stated on the label for those with allergies.		

Products like this cereal are in a class of processed foods that I consider the *ultimate AD/HD-provoking foods*. With our children eating these "foods" several times a day, as breakfast and as a snack, it's no wonder they cannot concentrate. Scrutinizing labels will become an important part of overcoming AD/HD.

Making Favorite Recipes AD/HD Friendly

Now that you have the basic outlines for planning the day's menu, I will show you how you can take any recipe and fit it into one of the grids. You are going to restock your pantry with the substitute products you will need to beat AD/HD. I will teach you how to make simple adjustments to favorite recipes so they can be used in my *30-Day Plan*. Let's begin by listing the substitutes you will use for some common ingredients.

The following table lists the nonapproved ingredient and its approved substitute for your newly overhauled pantry. You will find in some cases I have listed brand names for hard-to-find items.

RECIPE SUBSTITUTION LIST

INGREDIENT	SUBSTITUTION (look for brands in appendix 2)
Mayonnaise (contains eggs, egg yolks, sugar, calcium disodium EDTA)	Eggless canola oil mayonnaise. To reduce fat for dressings you can substitute soy yogurt mixed with mango chutney. See recipe on p. 198.
Margarine (contains hydrogenated fats, emulsifiers, artificial colors)	Homemade Sunshine Butter (recipe included) or nonhydrogenated margarine.
Eggs as binders in cooking	Energee Wonder Slim egg replacer. Most egg replacers have egg whites in them. It's the protein in egg whites that causes a problem.
Cornstarch or flour for thickening	Arrowroot powder, kudzu root or tapioca root powder, potato or sweet rice flour.
Orange juice	Grapefruit, lemon, lime, papaya, mango, pineapple, carrot, or vegetable juice, rice milk.
Raisins (if allergic)	Unsulfured dried cranberries, dates, figs.
Peanuts, almonds (only if you are salicylate sensitive), and their butters	Pistachios, cashews, walnuts, pecans, hazelnuts, sesame seeds and their butters. Sunflower and pumpkin seeds.
Salt	Use half as much as most recipes call for, or try Spike or other salt-free seasoning containing a blend of salt-free green herbs, dehydrated onion, chives, or garlic.

INGREDIENT	SUBSTITUTION (look for brands in appendix 2)
Baking powder	Rumford's baking powder does not contain aluminum; many standard brands do.
Sugar	Fructose, Fruitsource, honey, rice syrup, molasses, true maple syrup or maple sugar (one half cup per one cup of sugar), fruit concentrate syrup
Milk products	Soy milk, oat milk, pecan milk, almond milk (unless salicylate sensitive), brazil milk, filbert milk, cashew milk (cream substitute), soy cheese, soy yogurt, soy sour cream, rice cheese.
Grain (Flours)	Brown rice, white rice, sweet rice, kamut, spelt, millet, oat, rye, soy, quinoa, buckwheat, teff.
Grains (Whole)	Barley, kamut, millet, oats, rye, amaranth, quinoa, teff (see complete lists in appendices)
Chocolate	Carob (doesn't need sweetening).
Bouillon	Miso paste—light miso for chicken, medium miso for vegetables and fish, or dark miso for beef or other meats. Use Edward & Sons Miso Soup packets or other organic bouillon cubes and flavored miso pastes.

MAKING SUBSTITUTIONS IN RECIPES
What's For Dinner?

Most menu planning is done around the main meal of the day. There-fore, we will begin applying our schematics from chapter 15 here. Don't be concerned about what your child has eaten earlier in the day. Few of us are organized enough to have the whole day's menu planned ahead. You can decide what to eat for breakfast and lunch the day *after* preparing any of the three basic dinner schematics.

PART ONE—APPLYING THE TRADITIONAL MEAT, STARCH, VEGGIE (MSV) MEAL PLAN

Let's start with a delicious nutty chicken that your family will love. For adults, a creamy mustard sauce offers a nice tangy contrast to the chicken. Children will no-doubt elect to eat their chicken without the sauce. The original recipe contains too much fat, so we are going to modify the prepa-ration to reduce the fat. This recipe fits into the traditional MSV schematic.

PECAN-CRUSTED CHICKEN WITH MUSTARD SAUCE

INGREDIENTS AS THE RECIPE STANDS	INGREDIENTS TO SUBSTITUTE— AD/HD SAFE
1 cup pecans	
2 tablespoons cornstarch	2 tablespoons sweet rice flour, arrowroot powder, or potato flour
1 teaspoon dried thyme	
1 teaspoon paprika	
1½ teaspoons salt	1 teaspoon salt
⅛ teaspoon cayenne	
1 egg	1 tablespoon Energee Wonder Slim Egg Replacer
2 tablespoons water	
4 boneless, skinless chicken breasts (about 1¼ pounds total)	
3 tablespoons cooking oil	Do not add oil.
1 cup mayonnaise	1 cup nonfat soy yogurt
2 tablespoons grainy or Dijon mustard	2 tablespoons Dijon mustard, Westbrae or Tree of Life brands
½ teaspoon white-wine vinegar	½ teaspoon rice vinegar (milder), Nagano or other brand
½ teaspoon sugar	¼ teaspoon honey
2 tablespoons chopped fresh parsley	

Directions

1. In a food processor, pulse the pecans with the cornstarch (rice flour), thyme, paprika, ¾ teaspoon of the salt, and cayenne until the nuts are chopped fine. Transfer the mixture to a medium bowl.

2. Whisk together the egg (egg substitute) and the water in a small bowl. Dip each chicken breast into the egg mixture and then into the nut mixture.

3. In a large nonstick frying pan, heat the oil over moderate heat. Add the chicken to the pan and cook for 5 minutes. Turn and continue cooking until the chicken is golden brown and cooked through, 5 to 6 minutes longer. (Arrange the coated pieces of chicken on a rack in a broiler or baking pan. Bake at 375°F for 40 minutes.)

4. Meanwhile, in a small bowl, combine the mayonnaise (nonfat soy yogurt), mustard, vinegar, sugar (honey), parsley, pinch of cayenne, and the remaining ¼ teaspoon salt. Serve the chicken with the mustard dipping sauce.

Makes six 3-ounce servings

Comments: Apply this recipe to the MSV schematic and reduce the soy milk servings to one. We are using one soy serving in the preparation of the dipping sauce, and if you serve the grated carrot and apple or pineapple salad, you'll use another cup of soy yogurt.

See how easy it is! Now what about the starch and the vegetable? The pecan-crusted chicken can be served with mashed or baked potatoes or rice and a green vegetable (green beans). A grated carrot and fruit salad dressed with yogurt chutney dressing rounds out the meal. Here is a quick recipe for the dressing.

YOGURT AND CHUTNEY DRESSING

Ingredients

1 cup of nonfat or low-fat soy or rice yogurt
2 tablespoons chutney (contains some sugar but no additives)

Directions

1. Mix the yogurt and chutney
2. Add a little ground ginger, nutmeg, or cinnamon to suit your taste.
Makes 1 cup of dressing

Comments: This dressing makes a good substitute for mayonnaise dressings. It goes well on fruit salads or carrot and apple (or pineapple) salad. You can even use it on pancakes, hot cereal, or fruit for breakfast. The protein in the yogurt helps balance the sugar that's in the chutney. Just don't overdo it and start putting it on foods several times a day or even daily.

There are recipes for some other meals that fit into the MSV schematic.

BAKED FILLET OF SOLE WITH LEMON AND CAPERS

Ingredients
4 medium-size fillets of Dover sole, approximately 1 lb.
1 thin lemon slice for each fillet
½ teaspoon capers for each fillet
Mixed pepper blend, salt only if absolutely necessary.

Directions
1. Preheat oven to 350°F.
2. Wash fillets and pat dry with a paper towel.
3. Roll each fillet and place in a shallow baking dish. Top with a lemon slice and capers.
4. Cover the dish with foil and bake for 20 minutes. Use the pan juices over the fish or on top of each serving of rice. You can also thicken the juices slightly by mixing a little arrowroot powder paste into the juices and heating over low heat, while stirring constantly with a whisk.
Makes four servings, or more if you have very young children

Comments: This dish is quick and easy to fix. Serve it with steamed confetti rice, steamed spinach with nutmeg, and cooked acorn squash seasoned with pumpkin pie spice and a little bit of Sunshine Butter. (This is the sample I used in chapter 15 for the traditional Meat, Starch, and Vegetable plan.)

Variations
- You can also fix baked sole by using an egg substitute and a barley flour/ground almond mix, similar to the recipe listed for pecan chicken. Salmon is very good fixed this way and it contains more DHA. Salmon will require 25 to 30 minutes baking time.

CONFETTI RICE

Ingredients

I cup uncooked rice

I cup finely chopped vegetables (carrots; summer squash; celery; red, green and yellow peppers (or sun-dried tomatoes for the red color); parsley; mushrooms; nori or other sea vegetables. The idea is to select vegetables for a variety of color so the dish is bright and appealing. Look for orange, yellow, red, green, purple, etc.

Directions

1. Chop all the vegetables and set aside.

2. Bring 2 cups of water to a boil and add ½ teaspoon salt or Spike and I teaspoon olive oil.

3. Slowly add rice and return to a boil. Simmer for 20 minutes on very low heat.

Makes 3 cups, enough for 6 servings.

Comments: Any starch can be prepared this way. Ever think of adding vegetables to your mashed potatoes? Garlic mashed potatoes are a favorite in my family, but onions, mushrooms, or green veggies can be added as well. Mash the potatoes with the water, or you can add a little nut milk for a different flavor.

ROAST BEEF, PORK, OR LAMB WITH MASHED POTATOES AND GRAVY

This popular dinner doesn't need a recipe, but you will need to make a few adjustments. First of all, select the leanest cut of beef, pork, or lamb you can find. Don't salt the roast, but you can use pepper and spices of your choosing. For example, use bay leaves for roast beef, sage for pork, and garlic, curry, or mint for lamb. Roast at 325°F for 30–40 minutes per pound until desired doneness is reached. Or consult your favorite cookbook. Choose any of the vegetables listed in the menu plan food substitution list in chapter 15. If you like horseradish with your roast beef, choose the kind that's prepared with vinegar and salt only, not the creamed variety. Prepare the mashed potatoes using the suggestions I gave above. Use the following recipe for Basic White Sauce to prepare gravy. Just substitute some of the melted beef fat for the butter and the meat juices for the soy milk.

BASIC WHITE SAUCE

Ingredients

4 tablespoons Sunshine Butter, canola, or olive oil

2 cups soy milk (rice milk is sweeter and is desirable for some recipes)

¼ teaspoon salt

⅛ teaspoon pepper

2½ tablespoons sweet rice flour, arrowroot, or any whole grain flour other than wheat

Directions

1. Over low heat, melt butter in 1¾ cups of the soy milk.
2. Add salt and pepper to the warm soy milk mixture.
3. Make a smooth paste of the sweet rice flour and ¼ cup of the soy milk.
4. Add slowly to warm soy milk mixture.
5. Stir over low heat until thickened.

Makes 2 cups

Comments: I prefer using sweet rice flour over the other flours because it keeps the sauce from separating. It is easier to use than flour when making meat gravy because the paste can be added directly to warm pan drippings. Just be sure to adjust the amount of fat and juice you are using. Arrowroot can also be made into a paste and added directly to the hot juices. Arrowroot has the advantage of yielding a clear sauce, preferable for fish sauces, sweet-and-sour dishes, and vegetable sauces. Use 2 teaspoons arrowroot per cup of liquid. Clear sauces are flavored with miso, vinegar, honey, lemon, or natural juices from cooking seafood, chicken, or vegetables.

PART TWO—APPLYING THE ONE-DISH-MEAL (ODM) MENU PLAN

Most families are extremely busy today, and the traditional MSV plan doesn't work for most weekday dinners. Fortunately, recipes for one-dish meals that contain meat, poultry, or fish are easily prepared and share many similarities. This enables you to easily substitute favorite recipes into the basic ODM meal plan. Here is the plan and the number of daily servings of each food group accounted for in the menu plan for a seven-to-ten-year-old child. You can compare these with the menu plan for your age and gender from chapter 15.

STARCH 2 daily servings ½ cup each	PROTEIN/FAT 4 daily servings I ounce each	VEGGIES ½ daily servings ½ cup each	EMBELLISHMENTS freebees	ONE-DISH MEALS recipes serves 6 to 8
Rice Legumes Pasta Potatoes Bread	Fish Poultry Cheese Pork Lamb Beef Tofu Beans Split peas Lentils	Anything fresh, Any frozen veggie except corn, Sun-dried tomatoes	Salt, pepper, capers, pickles, green peppercorns, red, green, and chili peppers, lemon juice or zest, garlic, chives, onions, horseradish, mustard, ginger, mint, Tamari sauce	
EXAMPLES				
Fettuccini	Ground beef or turkey Grated cheddar rice cheese Canola oil	Chopped celery, carrots, tomatoes, tomato paste, spinach	Onion, garlic, salt, pepper, oregano, basil, thyme	Italian Beef and Veggie Casserole (recipe below)
Spaghetti squash Black beans	Pork loin Olive oil Parmesan cheese (soy or rice)	Tomatoes, celery, cabbage, zucchini, carrots	Onion, garlic, parsley, oregano, basil, chives, salt, pepper, chili powder	Old-World Minestrone Soup (recipe below)

The *Italian Beef and Vegetable Casserole* is a classic. Many variations of this basic one-dish meal are possible. I will give you some of them below.

ITALIAN BEEF AND VEGETABLE CASSEROLE

Ingredients
I cup finely chopped celery
½ cup finely chopped carrot
½ cup finely chopped onion

2 cloves of garlic, minced

¼ cup olive or canola oil

1 pound lean ground beef

¾ cup tomato paste

3 cups chopped tomatoes (Muir Glen, organic)

1 teaspoon salt (or less)

1½ teaspoon oregano

1 teaspoon basil

½ teaspoon thyme

10 ounces frozen chopped spinach or 4 cups chopped fresh spinach

4 ounces Arrowhead Mills Rice Fettuccini

1 cup grated Cheddar Rice Cheese

Directions

1. Sauté celery, carrot, onion, and garlic in oil.
2. Add beef and brown.
3. Add tomato paste, tomatoes, and seasonings. Simmer for 1 hour.
4. Cook spinach and drain well; add with noodles to sauce.
5. Turn into casserole. (You may cover and freeze at this time.)
6. Top with cheese before baking.
7. Bake at 350° for 20 minutes if warm, or 45 minutes if cold.

Makes 6 to 8 servings

Easy Substitutions for This Meal in the *30-Day Plan*

• The following dinners have similar nutritional content: *Chili with Beans, Hearty Bean Soup,* and *Ground Beef and Eggplant Moussaka.*

GROUND BEEF AND EGGPLANT MOUSSAKA

Ingredients

1 eggplant (one pound), peeled and sliced thinly

1 tablespoon olive oil

1 pound ground beef or lamb

1 onion, chopped

1 green pepper, chopped

2 cloves of garlic, crushed

2 cups tomatoes (Muir Glen, organic) or use fresh tomato slices, one for each
  eggplant slice

1 cup tomato sauce (Muir Glen, organic) or leftover pasta sauce

½ teaspoon salt

freshly ground black pepper

1 bay leaf
1 cinnamon stick or 1 teaspoon ground cinnamon
⅛ teaspoon ground allspice
1 cup cooked rice, or rice pasta, cooked

Topping:

1 cup soy or rice yogurt
2 teaspoons egg substitute
1 teaspoon lemon zest
1 teaspoon nutmeg

Directions

1. Brown the eggplant on both sides, using as little olive oil as possible
2. Meanwhile, sauté the beef or lamb, onion, green pepper, and garlic in a spray-coated nonstick pan
3. Add the tomatoes, tomato sauce, and seasonings, and simmer for 15 to 20 minutes.
4. Lightly oil a flat oblong or rectangular dish and layer the eggplant, rice (or pasta), and meat mixture.
5. Beat the yogurt and egg substitute together, add the lemon zest and nutmeg, and pour over the top of the layered casserole.
6. Bake in a 375°F oven for 30 minutes.
Makes 6 to 8 servings

Comments: If this is a little too spicy for your children, back off on the cinnamon, allspice, and nutmeg.

Variations

• If you like curries, substitute ground pork or ground turkey, or stay with lamb. Substitute ½ cup coconut milk and 1½ cups chicken broth or miso broth for the tomatoes. Use ginger and curry powder instead of cinnamon, allspice, and nutmeg. Eliminate the topping and serve the curry over hot steamed rice. Pass cashews, raisins, and green onions to be added at the table.

All hearty soups fit nicely into the ODM menu plan, as will vegetarian casseroles that combine legumes, tofu, and soy or rice cheese. If you don't use cheese, you can use the 4 fats and 1 protein it contains at another meal during the day. Here is an excellent hearty soup recipe.

OLD-WORLD MINESTRONE SOUP

Ingredients

¾ pound boneless pork loin or beef chuck, trimmed of fat and cut into ½-inch
  cubes
3 large garlic cloves, minced or put through a garlic press
1 medium zucchini, sliced
2 tablespoons plus 1 teaspoon olive oil (divided)
1 small spaghetti squash
2 carrots, sliced
1 onion, chopped
1 stalk celery, chopped
¼ head of cabbage, chopped
1 teaspoon each of salt, chili powder, dried oregano, basil, and chives
¼ teaspoon pepper
2 cups canned tomatoes (Muir Glen, organic)
½ cup fresh chopped parsley
1 2-cup- or 15-ounce-size can Great Northern or black beans

Directions

1. Brown pork until well done in a skillet with 1 teaspoon of olive oil.
2. Cover with water and simmer until tender, approximately 45 minutes.
3. In the meantime, pierce skin of spaghetti squash in several places and cook
in microwave on high until soft, 10 to 12 minutes.
4. When pork is done, place it in a soup pot and add the vegetables.
5. Cover with water, then add the spices, tomato juice, parsley, salt, and
pepper. Simmer on low heat until vegetables are very tender, approximately
1 hour.
6. Add the canned beans, 2 tablespoons of vegetable oil, and the cooked
spaghetti squash. Simmer another 15 minutes. Serve with grated soy or rice
Parmesan cheese.
Makes 12 servings

Comments: You can substitute other vegetables and use ½ cup of rice macaroni instead of the spaghetti squash. This soup tastes better the day after it's
made, and it freezes exceptionally well if you don't want leftovers.

Variations

- *Gingered Cabbage Soup with Pork and Potatoes.* Substitute 1 pound potatoes (3 medium) and 3 cups shredded cabbage for the carrots, celery, garlic,

zucchini, tomatoes, beans, and spaghetti squash. Use 1½ quarts boiling water flavored with 3 tablespoons medium miso paste, 2 tablespoons fresh grated ginger root, and 1 teaspoon lemon zest, instead of the spices listed above, to simmer the pork.

- *Turkey and Sweet Potato Soup.* Substitute turkey meat for the pork, 1 pound of sweet potatoes for the beans and spaghetti squash, and ½ pound of green beans for the tomatoes, celery, garlic, and zucchini. Make a broth of 1½ quarts water and light miso paste. Season with salt, 1½ teaspoons sage, and ¼ teaspoon ground pepper instead of the parsley, basil, oregano, and chili powder.

PART THREE—APPLYING THE STARCHY ONE-DISH-MEAL (SODM) MENU PLAN

Nearly every child I've worked with loves boxed macaroni and cheese dinners, but they are usually loaded with ingredients that can contribute to AD/HD symptoms. Here is a substitute for this classic favorite that they will love. We are going to use the same strategy we used for the construction of one-dish meals, except the starchy version uses more starch and less protein. Here is how it looks:

STARCH 2 daily servings ½ cup each	PROTEIN/FAT 4 daily servings 1 ounce each	VEGGIES ½ daily servings ½ cup each	EMBELLISHMENTS freebees	ONE-DISH MEALS recipes serves 6 to 8
Kamut or spelt macaroni	Soy or rice cheese Sunshine Butter		Mustard Salt and pepper	Macaroni and Cheese
Potatoes	Soy or rice cheese Soy milk, Sunshine Butter	sweet peppers	Salt and pepper Onions Roasted	Potatoes au Gratin

Both of the following recipes are adapted from originals and I will show you what to substitute.

MACARONI AND CHEESE

ORIGINAL INGREDIENTS:	AD/HD-SAFE INGREDIENTS:
½ pound semolina macaroni	½ pound spelt, kamut, or rice macaroni
2 tablespoons margarine	2 tablespoons Sunshine Butter or canola oil
2 tablespoons unbleached flour	2 tablespoons barley flour
2 cups milk	2 cups plain soy milk
I teaspoon prepared yellow mustard	I teaspoon prepared yellow mustard (Hain, Westbrae, or Tree of Life)
I cup grated cheddar cheese	I cup grated cheddar soy cheese
I teaspoon salt	I teaspoon sea salt
I teaspoon pepper	

Directions

1. Preheat oven to 400°F.

2. Pour 4 quarts of cold water into a large pot and heat on high until boiling.

2. Sprinkle macaroni into water and cook until al dente, approximately 10 minutes (see package directions).

3. To prepare sauce: Melt Sunshine Butter over medium heat. Stir in flour with a whisk, beating until smooth. Add soy milk and cook, stirring constantly with the whisk, until slightly thickened with no lumps. Remove from heat, and stir in salt, pepper, and mustard. Immediately stir in the soy cheese and set aside. Drain the macaroni and place in an oiled (olive or canola) casserole dish. Pour sauce over the macaroni and bake for 20 minutes.

Makes six 1-cup servings

Comments: Adding more seasonings can zip this dish up, but most children just want it plain.

Serve a mixed vegetable medley and a green salad with the macaroni and cheese or the potatoes au gratin recipe given below.

POTATOES AU GRATIN

ORIGINAL INGREDIENTS:	AD/HD-SAFE INGREDIENTS:
4 medium potatoes, peeled and sliced thinly in a food processor	
2 cups milk	2 cups plain soy milk
2 tablespoons butter	1 tablespoon Sunshine Butter or olive oil
1½ teaspoons salt	1 teaspoon Spike seasoning
Pepper	
½ pound cheddar cheese, grated	½ pound soy or rice cheddar cheese, grated

Directions

1. Preheat oven to 375° F.

2. Place alternating layers of sliced potatoes and soy cheese in a buttered (or oiled) 2-quart casserole. Dot with butter or oil, and sprinkle salt and pepper over each layer.

3. In the meantime, heat the soy milk over low heat until nearly scalding. Pour over the potatoes. Sprinkle a little paprika over the top.

4. Bake at 375° for 45 minutes, until potatoes are tender and the soy milk is absorbed. The soy milk will give the potatoes a slightly nutty flavor.

Makes six 1-cup servings

Comments: Potatoes au Gratin is extremely flexible. When you make the adjustments for meat and vegetables, this recipe fits the ODM meal profile.

Variations

• Add a pound of nitrate-free cooked sausage or ham, 1 cup of chopped sautéed onions, ½ cup of peeled roasted sweet peppers, or 1 cup of any combination of chopped veggies such as peas, more peppers, celery, carrots, or sun-dried tomatoes. Reduce the cheese to 3 tablespoons.

The SODM plan also allows you to introduce some other family favorites, such as pizza and tortilla-based dishes. Here are the necessary adjustments for pizza crust and corn or flour tortillas.

FLOUR TORTILLAS

ORIGINAL INGREDIENTS:	AD/HD-SAFE INGREDIENTS:
3 cups unbleached flour	3 cups barley flour
1 cup water	
2 tablespoons margarine or oil	2 tablespoons Sunshine Butter or canola oil
1 teaspoon salt	1 scant teaspoon sea salt

Directions

1. Mix the flour with water, salt, and oil, adjusting the quantity of water to make a stiff dough. The dough can be made ahead of time and kept in the refrigerator.
2. Knead the dough until the texture is smooth and elastic. Pinch off the dough into fifteen small balls. Flatten each ball between the palms of your hands and roll it out on a well-floured surface into a 7-inch circle. Keep the remaining balls in a bowl covered with a damp cloth to keep them from drying out.
3. Have an iron or other hot griddle ready. If your griddle is not the non-stick variety, spray ahead of time with a little olive oil cooking spray. When the bottom of the tortilla starts to brown, turn it over and cook the other side. During the browning process, pat the tortillas with a spatula to keep the bubbles that form from popping and tearing the tortilla.
Makes 15 tortillas

Comments: These tortillas can be used for tacos (MVS plan), bean burritos (SODM plan), or vegetable and chicken enchiladas (ODM plan).

Variations

• For "corn" tortillas, use 1 cup amaranth flour and 2 cups barley or other whole-grain flour.

Now let's tackle pizza. It really helps to have a bread maker, especially if your family loves bread. It will save you money in the long run, and it is more convenient to make AD/HD-approved breads from flour out of your pantry then to try and find the correct breads in stores.

PIZZA

ORIGINAL INGREDIENTS:	AD/HD-SAFE INGREDIENTS:
Dough:	
I tablespoon active dry yeast	I tablespoon preservative-free dry yeast
I ¼ cups warm water, I 10° F	
I teaspoon sugar	½ teaspoon honey
I ½ teaspoons salt	½ teaspoon salt
¼ teaspoon pepper	
2 tablespoons oil	2 tablespoons olive oil
3 cups unbleached flour	3 cups barley, rice, teff, or other whole-grain nonwheat flour
Sauce:	
2 to 3 cups prepared spaghetti sauce	Use the brands recommended
½ pound grated mozzarella, jack, or cheddar cheese	½ pound grated soy or rice mozzarella, jack, or cheddar cheese
¼ cup grated Parmesan or Romano cheese	¼ cup grated soy or rice Parmesan cheese
Toppings:	
sausage, pepperoni, hamburger, anchovies	Use nitrate-free versions, or tuna, herring, or sardines
	How about a veggie pizza?
Mushrooms, tomatoes, peppers	Onions, peppers, zucchini, mushrooms, olives, broccoli, green garlic

Directions

1. Preheat the oven to 425° F.

2. Dissolve yeast in warm water in a 2-cup glass measuring cup. Add the honey to "feed" the yeast, and stir to dissolve. Let rest 10 minutes or so, until the mixture bubbles to the top of the measuring cup. Stir in the salt, pepper, and oil.

3. Transfer to a large mixer bowl or food processor. Add flour a little at a time and work processor or mixer after each addition until the mixture is smooth and a soft ball forms and leaves the sides of the bowl. Turn out onto a floured surface and knead with your hands until it is smooth and elastic. The dough will be sticky. Using a bread maker? Follow the ingredients for your machine, making the appropriate substitutions.

4. Divide dough in half and roll out each piece to fit a lightly oiled 14" pizza pan. Fit into place and add the sauce and toppings.
5. Bake pizza for 20 minutes.

A family favorite is pizza made with pesto sauce in place of the tomato sauce. If you are lucky enough to get green garlic, it is fabulous. As more and more people discover this treat, stores are prompted to carry it. Green garlic looks like a large scallion, but the flavor is very mellow, though unmistakably garlic.

You have seen plenty of references to Sunshine Butter in the recipes I've given you. Children and grown-ups love this butter. It is soft and easy to spread and tastes wonderful. This recipe provides omega-6 and omega-3 oils, some vitamin E, natural vitamin A from the butter, beta carotene, fewer saturated fats, and no hydrogenated fats! Although butter is made from milk, it is less likely than milk to cause allergic reactions because it does not contain milk protein. Here is the recipe for it.

SUNSHINE BUTTER

Ingredients

1 pound unsalted butter (salted only if your family demands it)
1 cup canola oil
2 tablespoons DHA granules
½ dropper of natural liquid vitamin E
1 natural (not synthetic) beta carotene capsule (optional)
6 small (6 ounce) Pyrex custard cups or white ramekins

Directions

1. Let the butter come to room temperature.
2. Beat it in a mixer or food processor until it is creamy and soft.
3. Reduce mixer or processor speed, and slowly add the canola oil. Add the DHA granules or emulsion and carefully blend in. Add the vitamin E and squeeze the contents of the beta carotene capsule into the mixture. Pour the Sunshine Butter into the glass containers. Cover them carefully with plastic wrap, then with aluminum foil, and freeze. Defrost as needed; it only takes a few minutes. Keep refrigerated after use.

BREAKFAST

Breakfast is the most important meal you and your child can eat. Many adults skip breakfast, either because they are in a hurry to get out the door or because they don't feel hungry. There is a tendency for these individuals to choose sugary foods later in the morning, as energy levels sag. For someone with AD/HD, this can have devastating effects on mental performance. I explained in chapter 11 why eating sugar boggles the brain, and this isn't limited to those with AD/HD. Even if you don't think you have AD/HD, try my *30-Day Plan* and see what a difference in mental performance you will discover.

Adults and children will benefit from starting the day with a "power shake" made from high-protein ingredients. There is an endless variety of ways to fix this beverage. The power shake is a great pick-me-up in the afternoon, especially for children on their way to soccer practice or other after-school activities. My children and I were powered through countless swim meets with variations of the power shake. Be sure to include the digestive enzymes; they make all the difference in how this shake "sits on the adult stomach." Children can also have trouble digesting proteins, as I discussed in earlier chapters.

These recipes fit nicely into the meal-planning grid I gave you in chapter 15.

BANANA POWER SHAKE

Ingredients

6 tablespoons pineapple juice, or any *real* tropical juice without sugar (no orange juice)
6 tablespoons soy or rice yogurt
1 heaping tablespoon 85%—90% soy isolate protein powder
½ banana
1 tablespoon honey or 1 to drops stevia extract (optional)
1 tablespoon kerithin granules (optional)
1 teaspoon flaxseeds (optional)
2 digestive capsules
Ice cubes to thin to drinking consistency

Directions:

1. Blend all ingredients in a blender or drink mixer. Add ice cubes to achieve desired consistency.
2. You can use this beverage as a carrier for the dietary supplements.
3. Add contents of 2 digestive enzyme capsules to digest the protein.
Makes 1 shake

Comments: I recommend two power shakes a day for children, one in the morning and one mid-afternoon, after school. You will have to see how your child wants to take his or her supplements. Some prefer to swallow them with a swig of power drink. Others will handle putting the contents of the capsules into the drink. Adults usually drink one protein smoothie a day for breakfast. For women who are pregnant or lactating, a second one in the afternoon can be of benefit as well. Other adults and athletes like to drink a smoothie before working out.

Variations:

- *Vegetable Drink:* Use vegetable juice, carrot, tomato, or celery juice, either purchased or juiced from a home juicer if you own one. Use Organic Frog "Greens Today Protein Formula" for the protein powder. Make the drink a little zestier if you like with 2 drops of red Tabasco sauce and a squeeze of lemon juice. A teaspoon of miso paste can also be added.
- *Smoothie Drink:* Use any of the organically based smoothies you purchase ready-to-go. There are many excellent brands of these, usually found in the refrigerated section of your market. Pick either the green or soy protein powder to complement the flavor of the smoothie. Rice milk or apple juice can be used to thin the consistency.

BRAZIL-NUT BREAKFAST SHAKE

Ingredients

7 Brazil nuts
1 medium frozen banana (cut into chunks)
1 rounded tablespoon protein powder (Naturade soy)
1½ teaspoons carob powder
1 teaspoon maple syrup

Directions

1. Place 1 cup of cold water and brazil nuts into blender.
2. Blend on low for a few seconds and then turn to high speed.
3. Blend until smooth, scraping sides of container with a spatula if necessary.
4. Add frozen bananas, protein powder, carob, and maple syrup.
5. Continue to blend on high speed until consistency is smooth and creamy. Serve immediately.
Makes 1 shake

Variations

- Other nuts such as cashews, almonds, pecans, or walnuts can be used in place of brazil nuts. Other fruits, fresh or frozen, such as strawberries, mangoes, or melons, can be used in place of the banana.

WEEKEND BREAKFASTS

What about weekend mornings? You want a little variety, or maybe you are having company. Here are some great weekend breakfasts.

OAT-FLOUR PANCAKES

Ingredients

1 cup oat flour
2 teaspoons baking powder (Rumford's non–aluminum)
¼ teaspoon salt
2 teaspoons egg substitute
¾ cup liquid, half soy milk and half water
1 teaspoon honey or pure maple syrup
1 teaspoon vegetable oil

Directions

1. Stir oat flour, baking powder, and salt together in a medium mixing bowl.
2. Make a well in the dry ingredients and add the egg substitute, soy milk and water, and oil. Add the honey or maple syrup. Using a whisk, mix well.
3. Pour batter in spoonfuls onto a medium hot pan or griddle. Bake on one side until bubbles form on surface, then turn. Serve with 2 tablespoons real maple syrup and 2 teaspoons Sunshine Butter.
Makes 2 to 3 servings

Comments: Leftover pancakes can be individually frozen in plastic bags. You will want to serve a protein food with this to keep the balance correct. Suggestions include additive-free sausage, bacon, or ham. You can make your own sausage without the casings. See the recipe for *Breakfast Sausage.*

Variations

- The recipe makes delicious waffles also. Increase the canola oil to 2 teaspoons and use a Teflon-coated waffle iron. Two tablespoons of broken nut pieces, such as pecans, can be sprinkled on the batter just prior to closing the lid. Blueberries (3 tablespoons) also make a great change. Add 1 teaspoon of baking soda and use soy yogurt instead of soy milk for a "soured" flapjack or waffle. You will want to skip the Sunshine Butter on nut waffles. Try topping either pancakes or waffles with fresh berries or peaches and honey-sweetened rice yogurt.

BREAKFAST SAUSAGE

Ingredients

1 pound lean pork, turkey, chicken, or veal
1 clove garlic, put through a press
1 teaspoon fennel seeds
½ teaspoon chili powder

Directions

1. Mix meat with spices and shape into 8 patties.
2. Brown patties in skillet.
Makes 8 servings

Comments: This basic sausage recipe is one you can vary by changing the meats and spices you use. You can easily control the fat content by the meat you choose. Penzey's catalog, listed in appendix 2, offers several sausage blends. The sausage can be made ahead of time and frozen. Crumbled, it makes a great pizza topping or as an ingredient in a one-dish meal.

This next recipe is an AD/HD-approved variation on the popular frittata made with scrambled eggs and veggies.

BREAKFAST TOFU SCRAMBLER

Ingredients

1 pound Chinese-style tofu
2 tablespoons barley flour
1 teaspoon paprika
½ teaspoon garlic powder
1 teaspoon onion powder
½ teaspoon salt
¼ teaspoon curry powder
⅛ teaspoon pepper
1 onion, chopped
2 garlic cloves, minced
2 large carrots, grated
1 zucchini, cut in small pieces
1 cup chopped broccoli or cauliflower
½ cup snow peas, halved
½ cup chopped mushrooms

½ cup chopped spinach
2 teaspoons olive oil
1 teaspoon wheat-free Tamari

Directions
1. Cut tofu into slices, wrap in a paper towel, and gently press out excess moisture.
2. Mix spices and flour in a small bowl.
3. Sauté vegetables and garlic until partially cooked.
4. Crumble the drained tofu into the vegetables and continue to cook for 5 minutes.
5. When the vegetables are tender, add the flour mixture, the Tamari, and ½ cup of water. Stir well.
6. Continue cooking, stirring occasionally, until heated through. Serve immediately.
Makes 4 servings

Comments: This breakfast dish contains plenty of protein. You do not need to serve it with either the power shake or any meat.

In addition to these ideas I've provided, remember that leftovers make great breakfasts. For example, you can serve any of the three dinner plans for breakfast. You will simply have to make adjustments for the protein and carbohydrate servings according to which of the three dinner plans you are using. You will not have to use the power shake unless you are using the SODM plan.

What Do I Put in My Child's Lunch?

This is a very common question from parents. Luckily, parents can easily create exciting and tasty lunches that are healthy for their children and won't jam up their brain cells so they can't concentrate in the afternoon. These lunches promote clear thinking and a steady stream of energy throughout the afternoon and are therefore also suitable for busy working adults. Here are three examples.

Lunch 1:
   1 slice nonwheat bread (see appendix 2 for brands)
   Tuna salad, made with mayonnaise from the substitution list
   1 cup of strawberries
   1 serving vanilla pudding (see appendix 2 for brands)
   1 juice box (see appendix 2 for brands)

Lunch 2:

2 brown rice cakes spread with cashew butter and strawberry jam
Carrot and celery sticks
1 package Health Valley potato chips
2 date nut cookies (see recipe below)
1 juice box

Lunch 3:

Macaroni and Cheese (see recipe on page 207)
Raw baby carrots with tofu ranch dip
2 ounces mixed nuts, seeds, and dried cranberries (no peanuts or almonds)
1 cup cantaloupe cubes
1 cup vanilla soy milk

You get the idea. Just look at the substitution list for each of the food groups on page 195 and you can mix and match countless items for different, delicious lunch options for you or your child.

DATE NUT COOKIES

Ingredients

½ cup spelt flour
½ cup quinoa flour
2 tablespoons arrowroot powder
1 tablespoon cinnamon
½ cup chopped dates
3 tablespoons canola or flaxseed oil
3 tablespoons maple syrup
2 tablespoons lemon juice
1 tablespoon water
⅓ cup chopped walnuts

Directions

1. Preheat oven to 350°F.
2. Mix dry ingredients, dates, and walnuts together well in a medium mixing bowl.
3. Measure oil, maple syrup, juice, and water into a small bowl or measuring cup.
4. Add all at once to the flour mixture and mix quickly.
5. Place dough by teaspoons on a lightly oiled cookie sheet.
6. Bake about 9 minutes.
7. Remove from cookie sheet and cool on wire racks.

Makes 16 cookies

MAKING YOUR OWN MILK SUBSTITUTES

It's very easy to make tasty nut drinks and oat milk. Here is the basic nut milk drink.

NUT MILK

Ingredients

1 cup + 2 tablespoons nuts (blanched almonds, filberts, cashews or any nut
    other than peanuts)
1 tablespoon flaxseeds
2½ cups water

Directions

1. Put nuts, flaxseeds, and water in a blender or food processor.

2. Blend on high for about 2 minutes, or until the nuts are pulverized.

3. Strain the mixture through a fine mesh strainer or cloth tea strainer. Wire coffee filters work nicely for this, just set aside one for this purpose so it doesn't taste like coffee. You will have to press the nut mixture through the filter.

Makes 2 cups of milk

Comments: Flaxseeds add the essential omega-3 fatty acids (alpha-linolenic) and help thicken the mixture.

SWEETENED CASHEW CREAM

Ingredients

½ cup raw organic cashew pieces, unsalted
1 tablespoon Fruitsource, honey or maple syrup
1 tablespoon flaxseeds
2 cups water

Directions

1. Combine cashews with 1 cup of water, flaxseeds, and sweetener in a blender.

2. Blend on high until a thick cream is formed.

3. Slowly add the remaining water until thoroughly blended.

4. Strain only if it isn't smooth.

Makes 2 cups

Comments: Cashew cream is richer and thicker than other nut milks. You can control the consistency by how much water you add. Use this mixture as a substitute for cream. Natural vanilla or other flavoring can be added.

OAT MILK

Ingredients

⅓ cup organic rolled oats (old-fashioned kind)
2 cups of boiling water
Nutmeg, cinnamon, vanilla, or ginger to taste

Directions

1. Add the oats to the boiling water, cover, and cook on low for 2 to 3 minutes.
2. Set aside to cool.
3. When cool, mix in a blender with spice(s) of choice until the mixture is smooth and creamy. You can adjust the consistency by adding more water.
4. Chill before serving or blend in ice cubes for part of the water.
Makes 2 servings

Comments: This tasty beverage can be used as a beverage or as a base in any recipe that calls for milk or soy milk. The drink tastes better if it is allowed to sit in the refrigerator for an hour or more before consuming. Do drink it within a day or two, as it will mold quickly.

You will find dozens of additional tasty milk substitutes on the Internet at these addresses:

www.panix.com/~nomilk/nutmilks.txt
www.livingtreecommunity.com/recipes.html

DIPS FOR VEGGIES

CUCUMBER YOGURT DIP

Ingredients

1 cucumber, peeled, seeded, and cut into chunks
½ cup soy yogurt
1 teaspoon dill
¼ teaspoon lemon zest

Directions

1. Puree cucumber in blender.
2. Slowly add yogurt, dill, and lemon zest.
3. Blend until smooth or desired consistency.

Makes about 1 cup dip

Comments: You can adjust the thickness of this dip by how much yogurt you use. If you don't remove the cucumber seeds, the dip will have a thinner consistency. This cool summertime dip can also be used as a dressing on baked potatoes or vegetables.

MISO LEMON DIP

Ingredients

2 tablespoons dark miso paste
2 tablespoons boiling water
2 tablespoons rice vinegar
2 tablespoons lemon juice
1 teaspoon honey, or more to taste

Directions

1. Mash the miso paste until it is soft and pliable.
2. Add the hot water a little at a time to thin paste.
3. Add the vinegar, lemon juice, honey, and lemon zest.
4. Blend until smooth, and thin to desired consistency with hot water.

Makes about ½ cup dip

Comments: You can select the kind of miso your family prefers. The lighter the color of the miso, the milder the taste. Vary the amounts of honey and vinegar until you have the correct balance of sweet and sour.

Variations

• This dip recipe can be varied by adding minced onion, garlic, pickles, capers, or parsley.

Well, that does it for the recipes that should get you started on the *30-Day Plan*. Once you have a feel for the ingredients you should use and those you should avoid, I'm sure you'll be substituting to make new favorites from traditional recipes that you and your family will enjoy.

AD/HD-Provoking Additive Ingredients

Although they affect AD/HD sufferers most adversely, everyone should avoid the additives listed below. They are added to products to minimize spoilage and for other reasons, but they can cause problems with sensitive people.

Artificial flavors   Artificial flavors can come from purely synthetic or natural sources. Most food manufacturers do not list the exact ingredients of artificial flavors, which may consist of allergy-provoking substances. They can be irritating to the brain and nervous system.

Azodicarbonamide (ADA)   ADA is a conditioner used to bleach and mellow the flavor of flour for use in commercial breads. The allergic reactions to azodicarbonamide include asthma, cough, wheezing, and rashes.

Butylated hydroxyanisole (BHA)   This antioxidant preservative is used in food and beverages to prevent oxidation and retard rancidity in fats, oils, and oil-containing foods. A synthetic chemical, BHA can cause allergic reactions and in laboratory studies has been found to be weakly estrogenic in vitro. Dose-dependent European studies indicate a high incidence of cancerous and benign tumors in laboratory animals fed BHA. BHA is labeled as a possible carcinogen by the World Health Organization.

Butylated hydroxytoluene (BHT)   BHT is a prohibited food additive in England. Like BHA, BHT retards rancidity in foods such as cereals, potato chips, candies, oils, shortenings, frozen pork sausage, and many others. BHT may alter behavior and provoke hyperactivity in children. Published findings indicate BHT induces tumors in laboratory animals.

Calcium propionate   This preservative is used in breads, poultry stuffing, processed cheeses, and bakery products to inhibit mold. It may affect chemically-sensitive persons. This preservative is banned in Germany.

Calcium sulfite   Calcium sulfite functions as a dough conditioner and improves the baking quality of dough. Sulfiting agents such as this are known to cause mild to serious reactions in sensitive individuals.

Caramel color III   Caramel color III is used as a coloring and flavoring in baked goods, soft drinks, and ice cream. Toxicity studies demonstrate that caramel color III causes a reduction in total blood cell counts and disturbs immune functions in laboratory animals.

Casein   Casein is the principal protein in cow's milk and is used as a texturizer in ice cream, ice milk, fruit sherbets, frozen custard, coffee creamer, water-packed tuna, and many other foods. Casein may appear as sodium or calcium caseinate on labels and is the protein to which milk-allergic individuals are most likely reactive.

Citric acid   This multifunctional additive is used as a flavoring, neutralizer, antioxidant, sequestrant, curing and firming agent, and food brightener. Citric acid is not recommended for AD/HD children since it is extracted from any number of sources, including citrus fruits, beet molasses, and pineapple, or by fermentation of crude sugars. Also, allergy-sensitive children have an increased risk of a positive reaction to citric acid that may result in atopic dermatitis and gastrointestinal symptoms.

Cocoa (chocolate)   Chocolate contains methylxanthines and phenylethylamine, which can create an allergic response in some children. Cocoa may cause various symptoms of allergies such as wheezing and rash, particularly in children.

Corn oil   Corn oil acts as a texturizer, coating, and emulsifier in many processed foods, including bakery products, salad oils, mayonnaise, and margarine. Corn oil is not suitable for corn-sensitive individuals.

Corn syrup   Corn syrup is a derivative of cornstarch and is used as a sweetener and texturizer. It is used in snack foods, imitation dairy foods, candy, and many other foods; it is ubiquitous in processed foods. Corn syrup may cause allergic reactions and promote tooth decay.

Cottonseed oil   Cottonseed oil is used in a variety of products, from oleomargarines to nail-polish removers. Most commercial fried foods use cottonseed oil in its partially or fully hydrogenated saturated form. This highly saturated oil is known to cause allergic reactions. It can disrupt brain chemistry by interfering with essential fatty acid metabolism.

Dextrose   Dextrose, or corn sugar, is used as a coloring agent and sweetener in numerous prepared foods such as cookies, breads, and highly processed foods. Dextrose is a simple sugar with the same chemical composition as glucose.

Disodium inosinate   This flavor potentiator or intensifier is prepared from meat extract or dried sardines.

Disodium guanylate   A more effective flavor enhancer than sodium inosinate.

FD&C Blue No. 2 (Indigotine)   FD&C Blue No. 2 is an artificial synthetic coloring used in pet food, baked goods, candy, exotic teas, milk products, cereals, frozen desserts, and beverages. It contains sodium chloride or sodium sulfate. Although on the list of approved color additives, it acts as a sensitizer in allergy-sensitive persons. FD&C Blue No. 2 is banned in Norway. Tests on laboratory animals suggest that this additive may cause brain tumors, but this has not been proven.

FD&C Red No. 40   FD&C Red No. 40 or Allura Red AC is found in pastry, candy, pet food, sausage, soda pop, and desserts. The National Cancer Institute has reported that that p-credine, a chemical used in the Red No. 40 compound, is carcinogenic in laboratory animals.

FD&C Yellow No. 5 (Tartrazine)   Derived from coal tar, FD&C Yellow No. 5 (tartrazine) is America's second most popular food color. It is found in candy, pet food, soft drinks, cheese, crackers, and baked goods. FD&C Yellow No. 5 may cause allergic reactions, especially in aspirin-sensitive persons. It is reported that this common additive causes adverse reactions such as recurrent urticaria (a type of rash), coughing fits, swelling of mucous membranes, angioedema, and asthma. It is also implicated in hyperkinesis. In a double-blind placebo-controlled study reported in the *Journal of Pediatrics* (Nov. 1994), FD&C Yellow No. 5 caused behavioral changes, irritability, restlessness, and sleep disturbances in some children.

FD&C Yellow No. 6 (Sunset yellow)   FD&C Yellow No. 6 is used in bakery products, candy, and carbonated beverages. It induces allergic reactions such as purpura (skin reddening) or allergic skin hemorrhages in some children. In a recent study of forty-one multivitamin and mineral preparations, FD&C Yellow No. 6 was the most common dye in 46 percent of the preparations.

High-fructose corn syrup   High-fructose corn syrup is commercially produced from dextrose and is found in baked goods, cereals, salad dressings, ice cream, and other highly processed foods. It is quickly absorbed in the bloodstream and is not suitable for corn- or sugar-sensitive individuals. This is one of the worst offenders for those who suffer from AD/HD.

Hydrogenated or partially hydrogenated oil   Oil becomes hydrogenated by adding hydrogen, creating a stable, semisolid shortening. This procedure produces trans fats, which interfere with fatty acid metabolism. They have been implicated in several cancers, including that of the colon.

Hydrolyzed corn protein   Hydrolyzed corn protein is a protein made from corn that acts as a flavor enhancer. It is referred to as hydrolyzed vegetable protein (HVP), vegetable protein, or hydrolyzed plant protein (HPP). Although not specifically stated, hydrolyzed corn protein may contain glutamate (found in MSG) and cause adverse reactions in sensitive individuals.

Mono and diglycerides   A class of fats that act as emulsifiers by keeping oil and water mixed together, preventing rancidity in baked goods. Usually these fats are found in junk foods (baked goods, margarine, candy, peanut butter) that are high in fat, sugar, and flour. They are also used in coffee creamers/whiteners.

Monosodium glutamate (MSG)   This well-known flavor enhancer provokes reactions in some people that include headaches, migraines, asthma, and chest pain. It is often found in foods such as soups, salad dressings, restaurant food (unless otherwise specified), meat, baked goods, condiments, and numerous other products.

Natural smoke flavoring Natural smoke flavoring is used to flavor meat, fish, seasoned mixes, cheese, pizza, and dips, and is also used as an antioxidant to retard bacterial growth. Some natural smoke flavorings are produced by exposing yeast to wood smoke, which affects yeast- and additive-sensitive children.

Sodium acid pyrophosphate Sodium acid pyrophosphate is a slow-acting constituent in the leavening mixture for self-rising flours, mixes, and prepared bakery products. This preservative prevents discoloration in potatoes and sugar syrups. It is also found in canned tuna fish.

Sodium benzoate Sodium benzoate is used as a preservative (microbial control) in foods, including soft drinks, fruit juices, margarine, confections, pickles, and jams. Sodium preservatives add sodium to the diet and reduce the availability of potassium. Some reported reactions to sodium benzoate include recurring urticaria (rash), asthma, and eczema.

Sodium erythrobate Sodium erythrobate is a preservative used in pickling brine and accelerates color fixing in cured meat products. It is also found in baked goods and beverages.

Sodium nitrite or nitrate These toxic preservatives are used in meat processing to stabilize color, give a characteristic flavor, and inhibit the growth of dangerous botulism-causing bacteria. Sodium nitrite or sodium nitrate is found in ham, frankfurters, smoked fish, corned beef, and luncheon meats. Studies suggest that nitrites or nitrates can lead to the formation of nitrosasmines, which are potent cancer causing chemicals. Both children and adults should avoid fatty, salty foods that contain sodium nitrite or sodium nitrate.

Sodium phosphate Sodium phosphate is used as a texturizer, emulsifier, and sequestering agent (a preservative that prevents chemical and physical changes affecting flavor, appearance, texture, or color). Sodium and phosphate both interfere with the body's mineral balance. Of special importance is its competition with potassium and calcium.

Sodium stearoyl lactylate Sodium stearoyl lactylate acts as an emulsifier, plasticizer, dough conditioner, and whipping agent. It is found in baked products, liquid shortening, artificial whipped egg whites, frozen desserts, and pancake mixes.

Sodium tripolyphosphate (STPP) STPP is a texturizer and sequestrant. It is also used as a meat preserver to retain moisture in fish.

Sulfur dioxide   Sulfiting agents, a group of preservatives that includes sulfur dioxide, are found in many foods, from fresh fruits and vegetables to beer and wine. Inhalation of sulfiting agents destroys vitamin B_1 and can cause flushing, hypotension, asthmatic wheezing, and tingling sensations.

Tertiary butylhydroquinone (TBHQ)   This antioxidant contains petroleum-derived butane. TBHQ is used either alone or in combination with the antioxidant/preservatives BHT or BHA. The ingestion of one gram of this antioxidant has caused vomiting, ringing in the ears, delirium, and collapse.

Yeast   Yeast is a type of one-cell fungus that is a dietary source of folic acid. It is found in bakery products, hot dog and hamburger buns, pretzels, cheeses, barbecue sauce, and many other foods. Yeast converts sugar into alcohol and carbon dioxide in the fermentation process, causing allergic responses in some allergy-sensitive individuals.

Foods by Mail

If suitable foods are hard to find in your area, here is a list of mail-order sources for grains, baking mixes, nuts, and in some cases, complete meals. I have not tried all of them, but the ones I've tried delivered the product as ordered and on time.

Authentic Foods
1850 W. 169th St. #B
Gardena, CA 90247
(800) 806-4737
(310) 366-6938 fax
Web Site: pages.prodigy.com/AUTFOODS

Money orders, cashier's checks, and personal checks accepted. Does not accept credit cards. Shipment via UPS.

Wheat-free and gluten-free bakery flours, pancake and baking mixes, and natural flavors.

Diamond Organics
P.O. Box 2159
Freedom, CA 95019
(800) 674-2642
E-mail:
shop@diamondorganics.com
Web site: www.diamondorganics.com

No minimum order. Mastercard, American Express, Visa, and Discover
cards, money orders, and personal checks accepted. Shipment via
Federal Express overnight or 2nd Day, or UPS.

Organic vegetables, fruits, nuts, oils, dressings, soy dairy products,
flours, pasta, and fruit juices.

Ener-G Foods, Inc.
P.O. Box 84487
Seattle, WA 98124
(800) 331-5222
(206) 764-3398
Web Site: www.ener-g.com

Mastercard, American Express, Visa, and Discover cards, money
orders, and personal checks accepted. Shipment via UPS. Shipping
charges apply.

Wheat-free, gluten-free, low-protein, low-sodium, and lactose-restricted
diet products such as breads, baked goods, and soup mixes.

Gold Mine Natural Food Co.
3419 Hancock St.
San Diego, CA 92110
(800) 475-FOOD

Mastercard, Visa, American Express, and Discover cards, money orders,
and personal checks accepted. Shipment via UPS ground.

Organic, macrobiotic, and Earthwise products. Foods include oils, rice,
herbs, beans, cereals, noodles, and other products.

Once Again Nut Butter, Inc.
P.O. Box 429
12 South State St.
Nunda, NY 14517

(716) 468-2535
(716) 468-5995 fax

Money orders, cashier's checks, and personal checks accepted. Does not accept credit cards. Shipment via UPS.

Quality nut and seed products (butters), roasted nuts, certified organic products.

Pastariso Rice Innovations, Inc.
1773 Bayly St.
Pickering, Ontario
Canada LIW 2Y7
905-831-5433
905-831-4333 fax

Call corporate office for nearest mail order distribution center.

Kosher, gluten-free 100% organic rice products.

Penzeys, Ltd. Spices & Seasonings
P.O. Box 933
Muskego, WI 53150
(414) 679-7207
(414) 679-7878 fax
Web site: www.penzeys.com

No minimum order. Mastercard and Visa cards, money orders, and personal checks accepted. Shipment via UPS or Parcel Post.

Spices, curries, and seasonings, including salt-free blends.

Quinoa Corporation
P.O. Box 1039
Torrance, CA 90505
(310) 530-8666
(310) 530-8764 fax

Money orders, cashier's checks, and personal checks or COD accepted. Shipment via UPS ground.

Ancient Harvest organic quinoa grain, flour, flakes, and pasta.

Walnut Acres Organic Farms
Penns Creek, PA 17862-0800
(800) 433-3998
(717) 837-1146 fax
Web site: www.walnutacres.com

No minimum order. Mastercard, Visa, and Discover/Novus cards, money orders, and personal checks accepted. Shipment via Parcel Post and Express Delivery.

Organic meat, poultry, fish, pasta, flour, soups and soup mixes, rice, herbs, and spices, vegetables, fruits, dried fruit, nut butters, and supplements.

Vitamins and Supplements by Mail

If you can't find the vitamins and supplements locally that you need, here is a list of mail-order sources.

Bronson Vitamins and Herbals
1945 Craig Rd.
St. Louis, MO 63146
(800) 235-3200
Web site: www.jmedpharma.com

Mastercard, Visa, and Discover cards, money orders, and personal checks accepted.
$4.50 shipping charge. Shipment via UPS or U.S. mail.

Comprehensive selection of quality vitamins, minerals, nutritionals, and herbal supplements.

ChildLife Essentials
1348 Tenth St.
Santa Monica, CA 90401
(800) 993-0332
(310) 393-2135 fax

No minimum order. Mastercard and Visa cards accepted. Shipment via UPS.

Essential fatty acids, Friendly Flora/Bifidus, First Defense.

L&H Vitamins, Inc.
32-33 47th Ave.
Long Island City, NY 11101
(800) 221-1152
(718) 361-1437 fax
Web site: www.lhvitamins.com

Mastercard, Visa, and Discover cards, money orders, and personal checks accepted.
$4.50 shipping charge. Shipment via UPS ground.

Over 10,000 different premium brand vitamin products at discount prices.

Martek, Inc.
6480 Dubbin Rd.
Columbia, MD 21045
(800) 662-6339
410-740-0081
410-740-2985 fax
Web Site: www.martekbio.com

No minimum order. Mastercard, Visa, and American Express cards, money orders, cashier's checks, and personal checks accepted.
$3.00 shipping charge. Shipment via U.S. mail.

Neuromins DHA nutritional supplements.

Nutrition Express
P.O. Box 4076
Torrance, CA 90510
(800) 754-8000
(310) 784-8522 fax

No minimum order. Mastercard, Visa, and Discover cards, money orders, cashier's checks, personal, or company checks accepted. $4.00 shipping charge. Shipment via UPS, U.S. mail, or Express Mail delivery.

National-brand supplements including vitamins, minerals, herbs and miscellaneous products.

Resources

For the latest information on the ADD nutrition solution, visit www.thenutritionsolution.com. For information and facts about AD/HD, you can contact the following organizations:

American College of Preventive Medicine (ACPM)
1660 L Street, NW, Suite 206
Washington, DC 20036
(202) 466-2044
www.acpm.org

A national professional society for physicians committed to the practice of preventive medicine and health promotion.

American Preventive Medical Association (APMA)
P.O. Box 458
Great Falls, VA 22066
(800) 230-2762
www.healthy.net/APMA

Active grassroots network that advocates for health freedom.

Association for Applied Psychophysiology and Biofeedback (AAPB)
10200 W. 44th Ave., Suite 304
Wheat Ridge, CO 80033
(800) 477-8892
www.aapb.org

AAPB was founded in 1969 with the goal of promoting a new
understanding of biofeedback and advancing the methods used in this
practice.

Autism Research Institute
4182 Adams Ave.
San Diego, CA 92116
(619) 281-7165
www.autism.com

Founded in 1967, the Autism Research Institute conducts and fosters
scientific research designed to improve the methods of diagnosing,
treating, and preventing autism.

Feingold Association of the U.S.
127 E. Main St., Suite 106
Riverhead, NY 11901
(800) 321-FAUS
www.feingold.org

Founded in 1976, this national organization provides help for families of
children with learning or behavioral problems, including attention
deficit disorder. This nonprofit organization provides information about
the potential role of foods and synthetic additives in behavior, learning,
and health problems. A medical resource directory is currently being
designed.

Grandparents and Parents Against Ritalin (GPAR)
P.O. Box 157
Friendship, MD 20758
(800) 995-2010
www.chesapeake.net/vparker/

This organization's primary objective is to inform the public of natural
alternatives to Ritalin and offer financial support to those parents unable
to afford the natural alternatives.

Hyperactive Childrens Support Group (HACSG)
http://homepages.force9.net/hyperactive

A United Kingdom charity offering advice and support to hyperactive children and their families without reverting to drugs.

Learning Disabilities Association of America (LDA)
4156 Library Rd.
Pittsburgh, PA 15234
(412) 341-1515
www.ldanatl.org

Organization formed by concerned parents devoted to defining and finding solutions for the broad spectrum of learning problems.

Mothers & Others for a Livable Planet
40 West 20th St.
New York, NY 10011
(212) 727-4474
www.mothers.org

A nonprofit education organization working to promote consumer choices that are safe and ecologically sustainable for this generation and the next.

National Alliance for the Mentally Ill (NAMI)
200 N. Glebe Rd., Suite 1015
Arlington, VA 22203-3754
(703) 524-7600
www.nami.org

NAMI is a grassroots, self-help, support and advocacy organization dedicated to improving the lives of people with severe mental illness and their families.

Parents Against Ritalin (PAR)
National Headquarters
225 S. Brady, Suite 100
Claremore, OK 74017
(800) 469-5929
www.p-a-r.org

Parents Against Ritalin is an international nonprofit organization committed to providing natural health alternatives for managing AD/HD. A physician database is currently being designed.

The National Information Center for Children and Youth with Disabilities (NICHCY)
P. O. Box 1492
Washington, DC 20013
(800) 695-0285
www.nichcy.org

NICHCY is a clearinghouse for information on disabilities and issues pertaining to individuals (birth to age twenty-two) with disabilities.

The National Pesticide Telecommunications Network (NPTN)
www.pested.psu.edu/ai3.html

Information about pest control and regulatory agencies, U.S. Environment Protection Agency, and pesticide agencies.

HEALTH PROFESSIONAL REFERRAL RESOURCES

The following organizations have referral services and maintain a database of names of health professionals.

American Academy of Environmental Medicine (AAEM)
Box CN 100-8001
New Hope, PA 18938
(215) 862-4544
www.aaem.com

Over 400 physicians have grouped together to study and treat individuals with illnesses or health problems caused by adverse, allergic, or toxic reactions to a wide variety of environmental substances. The AAEM physician directory is included in the membership package.

American Academy of Pediatrics (AAP)
141 Northwest Point Blvd.
P. O. Box 927
Elk Grove Village, IL 60007
(847) 228-5005
www.aap.org/

Organization of 50,000 pediatricians dedicated to the health, safety, and well-being of infants, children, adolescents, and young adults. Provides physician directory and information about AD/HD for parents.

American Association of Naturopathic Physicians (AANP)
2366 Eastlake Ave. E, Suite 322
Seattle, WA 98102
(206) 298-0126
www.naturopathic.org

This association offers information on education and training in the field of naturopathy. Searchable database for naturopathic physicians (N.D.).

American College for Advancement in Medicine (ACAM)
23121 Verdugo Dr., Suite 204
Laguna Hills, CA 92653
www.acam.org/

Nonprofit medical society dedicated to educating physicians on the latest findings and emerging procedures in preventive/nutritional medicine. Searchable database for ACAM doctors.

American Holistic Health Association (AHHA)
P.O. Box 17400
Anaheim, CA 92817
(714) 779-6152
http://ahha.org

National clearinghouse for self-help resources promoting the enhancement of health through personal responsibility, considering the whole person, wellness-oriented lifestyle choices, and active participation in health decisions and healing. Searchable database for holistic practitioners.

The American EPD Society
141 Paseo de Peralta
Santa Fe, NM 87501
(505) 983-8890
www.best.com/~athene/epdns.html

Enzyme-potentiated desensitization (EPD) is a method of immunotherapy that involves desensitization with combinations of a wide variety of extremely low-dose allergens given with an enzyme that induces the production of activated T-suppressor cells. A list of 801 qualified physicians in the United States, England, and Canada is available through the American EPD Society.

TESTING LABORATORIES

The labs listed below do specialized analyses that are not generally available from a local medical laboratory.

Doctor's Data
170 West Roosevelt Rd.
West Chicago, IL 60185
(800) 323-2784

Mineral hair analysis for toxic metals and mineral balance; amino acid testing for neurotransmitter function

Great Smokies Diagnostic Laboratory
18A Regent Park Blvd.
Asheville, NC 28806
(800) 522-4762

Testing for parasites, yeast infection, digestive function, and mineral analysis

Spectra Cell Laboratories
515 Post Oak Blvd., Suite 830
Houston, TX 77027
(800) 227-5227

Blood cell and serum analysis for nutrient content; reveals specific deficiencies

REFERENCES

AD/HD Occurrence and Diagnosis

Biederman, Joseph, et al. "Diagnoses of Attention-Deficit Disorder from Parent Reports Predict Diagnoses Based on Teacher Reports." *Journal of the American Academy of Child and Adolescent Psychiatry* 32 (20) (March 1995): 315–22.

Cramond, Bonnie. "The Coincidence of Attention Deficit Hyperactivity Disorder and Creativity." The National Research Center for the Gifted and Talented (Yale University, University of Connecticut, University of Georgia, University of Virginia), March 1995.

Haislip, Gene. "Reading, Writing and Ritalin: An Address Before the Conference on Stimulant Use in the Treatment of ADHD." Washington, D.C., December 1996.

Hallowell, Edward, and John Ratey. *Driven to Distraction: Recognizing and Coping with Attention Deficit Disorder from Childhood Through Adulthood.* New York: Simon & Schuster, 1994.

Kwasman, A., B. J. Tinseley, and H. S. Lepper. "Pediatrician's Knowledge and Attitudes Concerning Diagnosis and Treatment of Attention

Deficit and Hyperactivity Disorders: A National Survey Approach." *Archives of Pediatrics and Adolescent Medicine* 149 (11) (November 1995): 1211–16.

Prior, Margot, et al. "Sex Differences in Psychological Adjustment from Infancy to 8 Years." *Journal of the American Academy of Child and Adolescent Psychiatry* 32 (2) (March 1993): 291–304.

Zametkin, Alan. "Attention-Deficit Disorder: Born to Be Hyperactive?" *JAMA (Journal of the American Medical Association)* 273 (23) (June 21, 1995): 1871–74.

Living with AD/HD

Cantwell, D. "Attention Deficit Disorder: A Review of the Past Ten Years." *Journal of the American Academy of Child and Adolescent Psychiatry* 35 (8) (August 1996): 978–87.

Holborow, Patricia. "Living and Coping with a Hyperactive Child." *Australian Family Physician* 15 (6) (June 1986): 798–99.

Girls with AD/HD

Faraone, S., J. Biederman, et al. "A Family-Genetic Study of Girls with DSM-III Attention Deficit Disorder." *American Journal of Psychiatry* 148 (1) (January 1991): 112–17.

Seidman, Larry J., et al. "A Pilot Study of Neuropsychological Function in Girls with ADHD." *Journal of the American Academy of Child and Adolescent Psychiatry* 36 (3) (March 1997): 366–73.

Boys with AD/HD

Sandberg, David, et al. "The Prevalence of Gender-Atypical Behavior in Elementary School Children." *Journal of the American Academy of Child and Adolescent Psychiatry* 32 (2) (March 1993): 306–14.

Satterfield, J. H., et al. "Multimodality Treatment: A One-Year Follow-Up of 84 Hyperactive Boys." *Archives of General Psychiatry* 36 (1979): 965–74.

AD/HD in Adolescence

Achenbach, Thomas, et al. "Six-Year Predictors of Problems in a National Sample: III, Transitions to Young Adult Syndromes." *Journal of the American Academy of Child and Adolescent Psychiatry* 34 (5) (May 1995): 658–68.

Ackerman, P. T., et al. "Teenage Status of Hyperactive and Non-Hyperactive Learning Disabled Boys." *American Journal of Orthopsychiatry* 47 (4) (October 1977): 577–96.

Lynam, D. R. "Early Identification of Chronic Offenders: Who Is the

Fledgling Psychopath?" *Psychological Bulletin* 120 (2) (September 1996): 209–34.

Satterfield, J. H., and A. Schell. "A Prospective Study of Hyperactive Boys with Conduct Problems and Normal Boys: Adolescent and Adult Criminality." *Journal of the American Academy of Child and Adolescent Psychiatry* 36 (12) (December 1997): 1725–35.

AD/HD Adolescents / Adults and Motor Vehicle Accidents

Barkley, R. A., K. R. Murphy, and D. Kwasnik. "Motor Vehicle Driving Competencies and Risks in Teens and Young Adults with Attention Deficit Hyperactivity Disorder." *Pediatrics* 98 (6) (December 1996): 1089–95.

Murphy, K., and R. A. Barkley. "Attention Deficit Hyperactivity Disorder Adults: Comorbidities and Adaptive Impairments." *Comprehensive Psychiatry* 37 (6) (November/December 1996): 393–401.

AD/HD in Adults

Biederman, J., et al. "Patterns of Psychiatric Comorbidity, Cognition, and Psychosocial Functioning in Adults with ADHD." *American Journal of Psychiatry* 150 (12) (1993): 1792–98.

Gualtieri, C. T., et al. "Attention Deficit Disorders in Adults." *Clinical Neuropharmacology* 8 (4) (1985): 343–56.

Manuzza, Salvatore. "Adult Outcome of Hyperactive Boys." *Archives of General Psychiatry* 50 (July 1993): 563–76.

———. "Educational and Occupational Outcome of Hyperactive Boys Grown Up." *Journal of the American Academy of Child and Adolescent Psychiatry* 36 (9) (September 1997): 1222–27.

Shekim, W. O., et al. "A Clinical and Demographic Profile of a Sample of Adults with Attention Deficit Hyperactivity Disorder, Residual State." *Comprehensive Psychiatry* 31 (5) (September/October 1990): 416–25.

Spencer, T., J. Biederman, et al. "Is Attention Deficit Hyperactivity Disorder in Adults a Valid Disorder?" *Harvard Review of Psychiatry* 1 (6) (March/April 1994): 326–35.

AD/HD in Families

Biederman, J., S. Faraone, et al. "Further Evidence for Family-Genetic Risk Factors in Attention Deficit Disorder." *Archives of General Psychiatry* 49 (September 1992): 728–38.

Comings, D. E. "The Role of Genetic Factors in Conduct Disorder Based on Studies of Tourette Syndrome and Attention Deficit Hyperactivity Disorder Probands and Their Relatives." *Journal of Developmental and Behavioral Pediatrics* 16 (3) (June 1995): 142–57.

Ernst, M., and A. Zametkin. "The Interface of Genetics, Neuroimaging, and Hyperactivity Disorder." *Psychopharmacology: The Fourth Generation of Progress.* New York: Raven Press, 1995, pp. 1643–51.

Faraone, S., and J. Biederman. "Do Attention Deficit Hyperactivity Disorder and Major Depression Share Familial Risk Factors?" *Journal of Nervous and Mental Disease* 185 (9) (September 1997): 533–41.

Hechtman, Lily. "Families of Children with Attention Deficit Hyperactivity Disorder: A Review." *Canadian Journal of Psychiatry* (August 1996): 350–60.

Zametkin, Alan. "Attention-Deficit Disorder: Born to Be Hyperactive?" *JAMA* 273 (23) (June 21, 1995): 1871–74.

AD/HD Sub-Types-Influence on AD/HD Expression

Faraone, S. "Attention Deficit Disorder and Conduct Disorder: Longitudinal Evidence for a Familial Sub-Type." *Psychological Medicine* 27 (2) (March 1997): 291–300.

Faraone, S., and J. Biederman. "Do Attention Deficit Hyperactivity Disorder and Major Depression Share Familial Risk Factors?" *Journal of Nervous and Mental Disease* 185 (9) (September 1997): 533–41.

———. "Is Attention Deficit Hyperactivity Disorder Familial?" *Harvard Review of Psychiatry* 1 (5) (January/February 1994): 271–87.

Seidman, L. J., J. Biederman, S. Faraone, et al. "Effects of Family History and Co-morbidity on the Neuropsychological Performance of Children with ADHD: Preliminary Findings." *Journal of the American Academy of Child and Adolescent Psychiatry* 334 (8) (August 1995): 1015–24.

Predicting AD/HD in Children, Based on Adult AD/HD

Biederman, J., S. Faraone, et al. "High Risk for Attention Deficit Hyperactivity Disorder Among Children of Parents with Childhood Onset of the Disorder: A Pilot Study." *American Journal of Psychiatry* 152 (3) (March 1995): 431–35.

Depression in Mothers of AD/HD Children

McCormick, L. H. "Depression in Mothers of Children with Attention Deficit Hyperactivity Disorder." *Family Medicine* 27 (3) (March 1995): 176–79.

Pregnancy Complications and AD/HD in Child

McIntosh, D. E., R. S. Mulkins, and R. S. Dean. "Utilization of Maternal Perinatal Risk Indications in the Differential Diagnosis of ADHD and UADD Children." *International Journal of Neuroscience* 81 (2) (March 1995): 35–46.

Allergies and AD/HD

Braly, James. *Dr. Braly's Food Allergy and Nutrition Revolution*. New Canaan, Conn.: Keats, 1992.

Egger, Joseph. "Psychoneurological Aspects of Food Allergy." *European Journal of Clinical Nutrition* 45 (1 suppl.) (1991): 35–45.

Marshall, Paul. "Attention Deficit Disorder and Allergy: A Neurochemical Model of the Relation Between the Illnesses." *Psychological Bulletin* 106 (3) (March 1989): 434–46.

Rapp, Doris. *Is This Your Child?* New York: William Morrow, Quill Books, 1991.

Allergy Effects on the Brain

Gaby, Alan R. "The Role of Hidden Food Allergy/Intolerance in Chronic Disease." *Alternative Medical Reviews* 3 (2) (April 1998): 90–100.

Philpott, William, and Dwight Kalita. *Brain Allergies: The Psychonutrient Connection*. New Canaan, Conn.: Keats, 1980.

Rogers, Sherry. *Depression Cured at Last*. Sarasota, Fla.: SK Publishing, 1997.

Treatment of AD/HD Allergy

Egger, Joseph, et al. "Controlled Trial of Hyposensitisation in Children with Food-Induced Hyperkinetic Syndrome." *Lancet* 339 (May 9, 1992): 1150–53.

Franklin, A. J. "Hyposensitisation for Food-Induced Hyperkinetic Syndrome" (letter). *Lancet* 341 (February 12, 1993): 437.

"Hyposensitisation in Children with Food-Induced Hyperkinetic Syndrome." *European Journal of Pediatrics* 151 (1992): 864–65.

King, H. C., and W. P. King. "Alternatives in the Diagnosis and Treatment of Food Allergies." *Otolaryngology Clinic in North America* 31 (1) (February 1998): 141–56.

Patriarca, G., et al. "Food Allergy in Children: Results of a Standardized Protocol for Oral Desensitization." *Hepatogastroenterology* 45 (19) (January 1998): 52–58.

Environmental Influences

Angle, C. R. "If the Water Smells Foul, Think MTBE." *JAMA* 266 (21) (December 4, 1991): 2985–86.

Mueller, D. K., and D. R. Helsel. "Nutrients in the Nation's Waters: Too Much of a Good Thing?" *U.S. Geological Survey Circular* # 1136 (1996): 12.

Raloff, J. "Picturing Pesticides' Impacts on Kids." *Science News* 153 (23) (June 6, 1998): 358.

Lead and AD/HD

Bellinger, D., et al. "Attentional Correlates of Dentin and Bone Lead Levels in Adolescents." *Archives of Environmental Health* 49 (2) (March/April 1994): 98–105.

Needleman, H. L., et al. "Bone Lead Levels and Delinquent Behavior." *JAMA* 275 (5) (February 7, 1996): 363–69.

Rimland, B. "Nutritional and Ecological Approaches to the Reduction of Criminality, Delinquency and Violence." *Journal of Applied Nutrition* 33 (2) (1981): 116–37.

Tuthill, R. W. "Hair Lead Levels Related to Children's Classroom Attention-Deficit Behavior." *Archives of Environmental Health* 51 (3) (May/June 1996): 214–20.

Parasites

Gershoff, S. N., M.D. "A Backwoods Parasite Heads for Town." *Tufts University Health and Nutrition Newsletter* 15 (6) (August 1997): 3.

Tan, J. S., M.D. "Human Zoonotic Infections Transmitted by Dogs and Cats." *Archives of Internal Medicine* 157 (September 22, 1997): 1933–43.

Over-Diagnosis of AD/HD

Jureidini, J. "Annotation: Some Reasons for Concern About Attention Deficit Hyperactivity Disorder." *Journal of Paediatrics and Child Health* 32 (January 1996): 201–3.

Diet and AD/HD

Burlton-Bennet, Jocelyn, and Viviane Robinson. "A Single-Subject Evaluation of the K-P Diet for Hyperkinesis." *Journal of Learning Disabilities* 20 (6) (June/July 1987): 331–35.

Carter, C. M., et al. "Effects of a Few Food Diets in Attention Deficit Disorder." *Archives of Disease in Childhood* 69 (1993): 564–68.

Conners, C. K. *Feeding the Brain: How Foods Affect Children.* New York: Plenum Publishing, 1989.

Muñoz, Kathryn, et al. "Food Intakes of U.S. Children and Adolescents Compared with Recommendations." *Pediatrics* 100 (3, pt. 1) (September 1997): 323–39.

Rimland, Bernard. "The Feingold Diet: An Assessment of the Reviews by Mattes, Kavale, Forness and Others." *Journal of Learning Disabilities* 16 (6) (June/July 1983): 331–33.

Stevens, Laura, et al. "Essential Fatty Acid Metabolism in Boys with Attention-Deficit Hyperactivity Disorder." *American Journal of Clinical Nutrition* 62 (1995): 761–68.

Treatment Options

Diller, Lawrence, M.D. "The Run on Ritalin." *Hastings Center Report* 26 (2) (1996): 12–18.

———. *Running on Ritalin.* New York: Bantam Books, 1998.

Hechtman, Lily, M.D. "Adolescent Outcome of Hyperactive Children Treated with Stimulants in Childhood: A Review." *Psychopharmacology Bulletin* 21 (2) (1985): 178–91.

Malone, M. A., and J. M. Swanson. "Effects of Methylphenidate on Impulsive Responding in Children with Attention-Deficit Hyperactivity Disorder." *Journal of Child Neurology* 8 (April 1993): 157–63.

Pincus, H. A., M.D., et al. "Prescribing Trends in Psychotropic Medications." *JAMA* 279 (7) (February 18, 1998): 526–32.

Safer, D. J., et al. "Increased Methylphenidate Usage for Attention Deficit Disorder in the 1990s." *Pediatrics* 98 (6) (December 1996): 1084–88.

Shaywitz, S. E., M.D., and B. A. Shaywitz, M.D. "Increased Medication Use in Attention-Deficit Hyperactivity Disorder: Regressive or Appropriate?" *JAMA* 260 (15) (October 21, 1988): 2270–88.

Wilen, T. E., J. Biederman, T. J. Spencer, and J. Prince. "Pharmacotherapy of Adult ADHD: A Review." *Journal of Clinical Psychopharmacology* 15 (4) (August 1995): 270–79.

Ritalin—Side Effects

Ahmann, P. A., et al. "Placebo-Controlled Evaluation of Ritalin Side Effects." *Pediatrics* 91 (6) (June 1993): 1101–06.

Barkley, R. A., et al. "Side Effects of Methylphenidate in Children with Attention Deficit-Hyperactivity Disorder: A Systematic, Placebo-Controlled Evaluation." *Pediatrics* 86 (2) (August 1990): 184–92.

Corrigal, R., and T. Ford. "Methylphenidate Euphoria." *Journal of the American Academy of Child and Adolescent Psychiatry* 35 (11) (November 1996): 1421.

Lipkin, P. H., et al. "Tics and Dyskinesias Associated with Stimulant Treatment in Attention-Deficit Hyperactivity Disorder." *Archives of Pediatric and Adolescent Medicine* 148 (August 1994): 859–61.

Wang, G. J. "Methylphenidate Decreases Regional Cerebral Blood Flow in Normal Human Subjects." *Pharmacology Letters* 54 (9) (1994): 143–46.

Ritalin—Safety Concerns

Rappley, Marsha, M.D. "Safety Issues in the Use of Methylphenidate." *Drug Safety* 17 (3) (September 1997): 143–48.

Food Effects on the Brain

Burlton-Bennet, Jocelyn, and Viviane Robinson. "A Single-Subject Evaluation of the K-P Diet for Hyperkinesis." *Journal of Learning Disabilities* 20 (6) (June/July 1987): 331–46.

Carter, C. M. "Effects of a Few Food Diets in Attention Deficit Disorder." *Archives of Disease in Childhood* 69 (1993): 564–68.

Coussens, Harriett. "Diet and Hyperactivity." *Journal of the Oklahoma State Medical Association* 77 (May/June 1984): 169–73.

Egger, Joseph. "Hyperkinetic Syndrome: Food, Brain and Behavior." Conference Proceedings, October 1996, Allergy Research Foundation. *Journal of Nutritional and Environmental Medicine* 7 (1997): 353–57.

Kaplan, Bonnie, et al. "Dietary Replacement in Preschool-Aged Hyperactive Boys." *Pediatrics* 83 (1) (January 1989): 7–17.

———. "Overall Nutrient Intake of Preschool Hyperactive and Normal Boys." *Journal of Abnormal Child Psychology* 17 (2) (1989): 127–32.

Rimland, Bernard. "The Feingold Diet: An Assessment of the Reviews by Mattes, Kavale, Forness and Others." *Journal of Learning Disabilities* 16 (6) (June/July 1983): 331–33.

Spring, Bonnie, R. J. Wurtman, and J. J. Wurtman, eds. "Effects of Foods and Nutrients on the Behavior of Normal Individuals." *Nutrients and the Brain* (1986): 1–47.

Sugar and AD/HD

Girardi, N. L., et al. "Blunted Catecholamine Responses After Glucose Ingestion in Children with Attention Deficit Disorder." *Pediatric Research* 38 (4) (October 1995): 539–42.

Hoover, D. W., and R. Milich. "Effects of Sugar Ingestion Expectancies on Mother-Child Interactions." *Journal of Abnormal Child Psychology* 22 (4) (August 1994): 501–15.

Murry, R. K., et al. "Insulin Effects on Glucose, Lipid and Protein Metabolism." *Harper's Biochemistry*, 22nd ed. Norwalk, Conn.: Appleton & Lange, 1990, pp. 534–45.

Roshon, M. D., and R. L. Hagen. "Sugar Consumption, Locomotion, Task Orientation, and Learning in Preschool Children." *Journal of Abnormal Child Psychology* 17 (3) (June 1989): 349–57.

Wender, E. H., and M. V. Solanto. "Effects of Sugar on Aggressive and Inattentive Behavior in Children with Attention Deficit Disorder with Hyperactivity and Normal Children." *Pediatrics* 88 (5) (November 1991): 960–66.

Wolraich, M. L., et al. "The Effects of Sugar on Behavior or Cognition in Children: A Meta Anaylsis." *JAMA* 274 (20) (November 22–29, 1995): 1617–21.

Food Additives and AD/HD

Boris, Marvin, and Francine Mandel. "Foods and Additives are Common Causes of Attention Deficit Hyperactive Disorder in Children." *Annals of Allergy* 72 (5) (1993): 462–67.

Rowe, Katherine. "Synthetic Food Colorings and Hyperactivity: A Double-Blind Crossover Study." *Australian Paediatric Journal* 24 (1988): 143–47.

Rowe, Katherine, and Kenneth Rowe. "Synthetic Food Coloring and Behavior: A Dose Response Effect in a Double-Blind, Placebo-Controlled, Repeated-Measures Study." *Journal of Pediatrics* 125 (1994): 691–98.

Ward, Neil. "Assessment of Chemical Factors in Relation to Child Hyperactivity." Conference Proceedings, October 1996, Allergy Research Foundation. *Journal of Nutritional and Environmental Medicine* 7 (1997): 333–42.

Wender, Esther, M.D. "The Food Additive-Free Diet in the Treatment of Behavior Disorders: A Review." *Developmental and Behavioral Pediatrics* 7 (1) (February 1986): 35–42.

Aspartame

Pardridge, William. "Potential Effects of the Dipeptide Sweetener Aspartame on the Brain." *Nutrition and the Brain* 7 (1986): 199–241.

Acesulfame K

Bertorelli, A. M. "Review of the Present and Future Use of Non-nutritive Sweeteners." *Diabetes Education* 16 (5) (September 1990): 415–22.

Mukherjee, A., and J. Chakrabarti. "In Vivo Cytogenetic Studies on Mice Exposed to Acesulfame K: A Non-nutritive Sweetener." *Food Chemical Toxicology* 35 (12) (December 1997): 1177–79.

Schiffman, S. S., et al. "Bitterness of Sweeteners as a Function of Concentration." *Brain Research Bulletin* 36 (5) (1995): 505–13.

Sucralose

Atkinson, H. G., ed. "A New Substitute for Sugar." *Health News* (Massachusetts Medical Society) (May 1998): 5.

Knight, I. "The Development and Applications of Sucralose, a New High-Intensity Sweetener." *Canadian Journal of Physiology and Pharmacology* 72 (4) (April 1994): 435–39.

Mezitis, N. H., et al. "Glycemic Effect of a Single High Oral Dose of the Novel Sweetener Sucralose in Patients with Diabetes." *Diabetes Care* 19 (9) (September 1996): 1005.

AD/HD and Elimination / Provocation of Foods and Additives

Carter, C. M., et al. "Effects of a Few Food Diets in Attention Deficit Disorder." *Archives of Disease in Childhood* 69 (1983): 564–68.

Egger, J., C. Carter, J. Soothill, and J. Wilson. "Oligoantigenic Diet Treatment of Children with Epilepsy and Migraine." *Journal of Pediatrics* 114 (1989): 51–58.

Egger, J., et al. "Controlled Trial of Oligoantigenic Treatment in the Hyperkinetic Syndrome." *Lancet* (March 9, 1985): 540–45.

Schmidt, M. H., et al. "Does Oligoantigenic Diet Influence Hyperactive / Conduct-Disordered Children: A Controlled Trial." *European Child and Adolescent Psychiatry* 6 (1997): 88–95.

How the Brain Works

Ackerman, Sandra. "From Perception to Attention." *Discovering the Brain*. Washington, D.C.: National Academy Press, 1992, pp. 104–22.

Crawford, Michael, et al. "Nutrition and Neurodevelopmental Disorders." *Nutrition and Health* 9 (1993): 81–97.

Ganong, William, ed. "Synaptic and Junctional Transmission." *Review of Medical Physiology*. Grosse Point, Mich.: Appleton and Lange, 1993, pp. 74–102.

Fats, Fatty Acids, and AD/HD

Arnold, E. L., et al. "Potential Link Between Dietary Intake of Fatty Acids and Behavior: Pilot Exploration of Serum Lipids in Attention-Deficit Hyperactivity Disorder." *Journal of Child and Adolescent Psychopharmacology* 4 (3) (1994): 171–82.

Bazan, Nicolas G., R. J. Wurtman, and J. J. Wurtman, eds. "Supply of n-3 Polyunsaturated Fatty Acids and Their Significance in the Central Nervous System." *Nutrition and the Brain* 8 (1984): 1–22.

Bourre, J. M., et al. "Structural and Functional Importance of Dietary Polyunsaturated Fatty Acids in the Nervous System." *Advances in Experimental Biology* 318 (1992): 211–29.

Katsuki, Hiroshi, and Shoki Okuda. "Arachidonic Acid as a Neurotoxic and Neurotrophic Substance." *Progress in Neurobiology* 46 (1995): 607–36.

Stevens, Laura, et al. "Essential Fatty Acid Metabolism in Boys with Attention-Deficit Hyperactivity Disorder." *American Journal of Clinical Nutrition* 62 (1995): 761–68.

———. "Omega-3 Fatty Acids in Boys with Behavior, Learning and Health Problems." *Physiology and Behavior* 59 (4/5) (1996): 915–20.

Vision and DHA

Birch, Eileen, et al. "Breast-Feeding and Optimal Visual Development."
Journal of Pediatric Ophthalmology and Strabismus 30 (1993): 330–38.

———. "Dietary Essential Fatty Acid Supply and Visual Acuity
Development." *Investigative Ophthalmology and Visual Science* 33 (11)
(October 1992): 3242–53.

Connor, W. E., et al. "Essential Fatty Acids: The Importance of *n*-3
Fatty Acids in the Retina and Brain." *Nutrition Reviews* 11 (April 1992):
21–29.

Essential Fatty Acids and Psychiatric Disorders

Hamazaki, Tomohito, et al. "The Effect of Docosahexaenoic Acid on
Aggression in Young Adults." *Journal of Clinical Investigation* 97 (1996):
1129–33.

Hibbeln, J. R., and N. Salem, Jr. "Dietary Polyunsaturated Fatty Acids
and Depression: When Cholesterol Does Not Satisfy." *American
Journal of Clinical Nutrition* 62 (1995): 1–9.

Essential Fatty Acids and Infant Nutrition

Birch, D. G., et al. "Retinal Development in Very-Low-Birth-Weight
Infants Fed Diets Differing in Omega-3 Fatty Acids." *Investigative
Ophthalmology and Vision Science* 33 (8) (July 1992): 2365–76.

Carlson, S. E., and S. H. Werkman. "A Randomized Trial of Visual
Attention of Preterm Infants Fed Docosahexaenoic Acid Until Two
Months." *Lipids* 31 (1) (January 1996): 85–90.

Crawford, Michael. "The Role of Essential Fatty Acids in Neural
Development: Implications for Prenatal Nutrition." *American Journal
of Clinical Nutrition*, suppl. (1993): 703S–10S.

Food and Agricultural Organization (FAO) / World Health Organization
(WHO). "Lipids and Early Development." Joint FAO/WHO Expert
Consultation on Fats and Oils in Human Nutrition. *Nutrition Review*
53 (7) (July 1995): 202–5.

Gibson, R. A., et al. "Effect of Dietary Docosahexaenoic Acid on Brain
Composition and Neural Function in Term Infants." *Lipids*, suppl.
(March 1996): S177–81.

Hoffman, Dennis, et al. "Effects of Supplementation with ω3 Long-
Chain Polyunsaturated Fatty Acids on Retinal and Cortical Development
in Premature Infants." *American Journal of Clinical Nutrition* 57, suppl.
(1993): 807S–12S.

Makrides, M. "Are Long-Chain Polyunsaturated Fatty Acids Essential
Nutrients in Infancy?" *Lancet* 345 (1995): 1463–68.

Uauy, R., M.D., et al. "Visual and Brain Function Measurements in Studies of n-3 Fatty Acid Requirments of Infants." *Journal of Pediatrics* 120, suppl. (1992): S168–80.

Werkman, S. H. "A Randomized Trial of Visual Attention of Preterm Infants Fed Docosahexaenoic Acid Until Nine Months." *Lipids* 31 (1) (January 1997): 91–97.

Breast Feeding versus Bottle Feeding Outcomes

Cant, Andrew, Janet Shay, and David Horrobin. "The Effect of Maternal Supplementation with Linolenic and Gammalinolenic Acids on the Fat Composition and Content of Human Milk: A Placebo-Controlled Trial." *Journal of Nutrition Science and Vitaminology* 37 (1991): 573–79.

Greenwood, Carol, and Rosemary Craig. "Dietary Influences on Brain Function: Implications During Periods of Neuronal Maturation." *Current Topics in Nutrition and Disease* 16 (1987): 159–216.

Lanting, C. I., et al. "Neurological Differences Between 9-Year-Old Children Fed Breast-Milk or Formula-Milk as Babies." *Lancet* 344 (1994): 1319–22.

Lucas, A., et al. "Breast Milk and Subsequent Intelligence Quotient in Children Born Preterm." *Lancet* 339 (1992): 261–64.

Wilson, A. C. "Relation of Infant Diet to Childhood Health: Seven-Year Follow-Up of Cohort of Children in Dundee Infant Feeding Study." *British Medical Journal* 316 (7124) (January 3, 1998): 21–25.

Essential Fatty Acids in Learning Disabilities

Stordy, Jacqueline. "Benefit of Docosahexaenoic Acid Supplements to Dark Adaption in Dyslexics" (letter). *Lancet* 346 (1995): 385.

———. "Essential Fatty Acids (EFAs) and Learning Disorders." Unpublished.

———. "Review of Literature on Dyslexia." Unpublished.

Minerals and Brain Function

Shils, Maurice, M.D., ed. *Modern Nutrition in Health and Disease*, 8th ed. Philadelphia: Lea & Febiger, 1994, pp. 144–286.

Zinc and AD/HD

Arnold, E. L., and N. A. Votolato. "Does Hair Zinc Predict Amphetamine Improvement of ADD/Hyperactivity?" *International Journal of Neuroscience* 50 (1990): 103–7.

Arnold, E. L., et al. "Potential Link Between Dietary Intake of Fatty Acids and Behavior: Pilot Exploration of Serum Lipids in Attention-

Deficit Hyperactivity Disorder." *Journal of Child and Adolescent Psychopharmacology* 4 (3) (1994): 171–82.

Ashmead, H. D., et al. "The Intestinal Absorption of Dipeptide-Like Chelates as Small Peptides." *Intestinal Absorption of Metal Ions and Chelates.* Springfield, Ill.: Charles C. Thomas, 1985, pp. 171–72.

Bekaroğlu, Mehmet, et al. "Relationships Between Serum Free Fatty Acids and Zinc, and Attention Deficit Hyperactivity Disorder: A Research Note." *Journal of Child Psychiatry* 37 (2) (1996): 225–27.

Fortes, C., et al. "Zinc Supplementation and Plasma Lipid Peroxides in an Elderly Population." *European Journal of Clinical Nutrition* 51 (1997): 97–101.

Pfeiffer, Carl, M.D., Ph.D. "Zinc as an Essential Mineral." *Mental and Elemental Nutrients.* New Canaan, Conn.: Keats, 1975, pp. 223–27.

Smith, Q. R. "Regulation of Metal Uptake and Distribution Within the Brain." *Nutrition and the Brain,* vol. 8. New York: Raven Press, 1990, pp. 29–31.

Stohs, S. J., and D. Bagchi. "Oxidative Mechanisms in the Toxicity of Metal Ions." *Free Radical Biology and Medicine* 18 (2) (1995): 321–36.

Toren, Paz. "Zinc Deficiency in Attention-Deficit Hyperactivity Disorder." *Biological Psychiatry* 40 (1996): 1308–10.

Magnesium and AD/HD

Kozielec, T., and B. Starobrat-Hermelin. "Assessment of Magnesium Levels in Children with Attention Deficit Hyperactivity Disorder (ADHD)." *Magnesium Research* 10 (2) (1997): 143–48.

Schmidt, M. E., et al. "Effect of Dextroamphetamine and Methylphenidate on Calcium and Magnesium Concentration in Hyperactive Boys." *Psychiatry Research* 54 (2) (November 1995): 199–210.

Starobrat-Hermelin, B., and T. Kozielec. "The Effects of Magnesium Physiological Supplementation on Hyperactivity in Children with Attention Deficit Hyperactivity Disorder (ADHD). Positive Response to Magnesium Oral Loading Test." *Magnesium Research* 10 (2) (1997): 149–56.

Other Trace Minerals

Mehansho, H. "Bioavailability and Efficacy of Iron from Ferrochel." *Proceedings of the International Conference on Human Nutrition,* January 24–25, 1998, Salt Lake City, Utah, p. 83.

Pollitt, E., and E. Metallinos-Katsarua. "Iron Deficiency and Behavior." *Nutrition and the Brain,* vol. 8. New York: Raven Press, 1990, pp. 29–31, 115–37.

Vahter, M., et al. "Concentrations of Copper, Zinc and Selenium in

Brain and Kidney of Second Trimester Fetuses and Infants." *Journal of Trace Elements in Medicine and Biology* 11 (4) (December 1997): 215–22.

Vitamin C and Co-Factor

Blazsó, G. "Edema Inhibiting Effect of Procyanidin." *Acta Physiologica Academiae Scientiarum Hungaricase* 56 (2) (February 1980): 235–40.

Blazsó, G., et al. "Antiinflammatory and Superoxide Radical Scavenging Activities of a Procyanidins Containing Extract from the Bark of *Pinus pinaster* sol. and Its Fractions." *Pharmacology Letters* 3 (1994): 217–20.

Cahn, J., and M. G. Borzeix. "Effects Observed on Brain Chemistry Changes Secondary to Multiple Infarction." Sem Hospital, *Paris Bulletin* (July 7, 1983).

Corbe, B., et al. "Study of the Effect of OPC (Endotelon) on Light and Circulation in the Choroid (Layer of the Eye)." *French Journal of Ophthalmology* 11 (5) (1988): 453–60.

Facino, M. R., et al. "Free Radical Scavenging Action and Anti-Enzyme Activity of Procyanidines from *Vitis vinifera*." *Arzneimittel-Forshung Drug Research* 44 (1) (1994): 592–601.

Passwater, R. A. "A Report on Attention Deficit Disorder." The Second International Pycnogenol Symposium, Biarritz, France, May 1995, pp. 132–38.

Robert, G., et al. "Action of Procyanidolic Oligomers on Vascular Permeability: A Study by Quantitative Morphology." *Biological Pathology* 38 (6) (1990): 608–16.

Roger, C. R. "The Nutritional Incidence of Flavonoids: Some Physiological and Metabolic Considerations." *Experientia* 44 (9) (September 15, 1988): 725–804.

Rohdewal, P. "Pycnogenol." *Flavonoids in Health and Disease.* C. A. Rice-Evans, and L. Packer, eds. New York: Marcel Dekker, 1998, pp. 405–19.

Vitamins and AD/HD

Anderson, G. H., and J. L. Johnston. "Nutrient Control of Brain Neurotransmitter Synthesis and Function." *Canadian Journal of Physiology and Pharmacology* 61 (3) (March 1983): 271–81.

Bernstein, Al. "Vitamin B_6 in Clinical Neurology." *Annals of the New York Academy of Sciences* 585 (1990): 250–60.

Brase, D. A., and H. H. Loh. "Possible Role of 5-Hydroxythrytamine in Minimal Brain Dysfunction." *Life Sciences* 16 (1975): 1005–16.

Coleman, M., et al. "A Preliminary Study of the Effect of Pyridoxine Administration in a Subgroup of Hyperkinetic Children: A Double-

Blind Crossover Comparison with Methylphenidate." *Biological Psychiatry* 14 (5) (1979): 741–51.

Pfeiffer, Carl, M.D. *Mental and Elemental Nutrients.* New Canaan, Conn.: Keats, 1975.

Rimland, Bernard. "Controversies in the Treatment of Autistic Children: Vitamin and Drug Therapy." *Journal of Child Neurology* 3, suppl. (1988): S68–78.

The 30-Day Plan

Calvo, Patricia, ed. *The Wellness Nutrition Counter.* University of California, Berkeley, and New York: Rebus, 1997, pp. 225–309, 309–429.

Goldfinger, S. E., ed. "Deciphering the Latest Report on Trans-Fats." *Harvard Health Letter* 23 (4) (February 1998): 3.

Robb-Nicholson, C., M.D., ed. "Dietary Fat Reconsidered." *Harvard Women's Health Letter* 5 (7) (1998): 6.

Shils, M., J. Olson, and M. Shike. *Modern Nutrition in Health and Disease,* 8th ed., vol. 2. Philadelphia: Lea & Febiger, 1994, p. A-15.

Pantry Management and Eating Out

Calvo, Patricia, ed. *The Wellness Nutrition Counter.* University of California, Berkeley, and New York: Rebus, 1997, pp. 225–309, 309–429.

Phytonutrient Content of Foods—Disease Prevention

Albertazzi, P., et al. "The Effect of Dietary Soy Supplementation on Hot Flushes." *Obstetrics and Gynecology* 91 (1998): 6–11.

Ingram, D., et al. "Case Controlled Study of Phytoestrogens and Breast Cancer." *Lancet* 350 (October 1997): 990–94.

Key, T. A., et al. "A Case Controlled Study of a Diet and Prostate Cancer." *British Journal of Cancer* 76 (1997): 678–87.

Rice-Evans, Catherine. "Antioxidant Activities of Carotenes and Xanthophylls." *FEBS Letters* 384 (April 22, 1996): 240–42.

Williams, J. K. "Soy Isoflavones Enhance Coronary Vascular Activity in Atherosclerotic Macaques." *Fertility and Sterility* 67 (January 1997): 148–54.

INDEX

Page numbers in italics indicate boxed text. Italic *f* after a number indicates illustration; *t*, table.